Living with Learning Disabilities, Dying with Cancer

Thirteen Personal Stories

Irene Tuffrey-Wijne

Foreword by Professor Sheila Hollins

Jessica Kingsley *Publishers*
London and Philadelphia

First published in 2010
by Jessica Kingsley Publishers
73 Collier Street
London N1 9BE, UK
and
400 Market Street, Suite 400
Philadelphia, PA 19106, USA

www.jkp.com

Printed digitally since 2013

Library of Congress Cataloging in Publication Data

Tuffrey-Wijne, Irene, 1963-
Living with learning disabilities, dying with cancer : thirteen personal stories / Irene Tuffrey-Wijne ; foreword by Sheila Rollins.
p. cm.
Includes bibliographical references and index.
ISBN 978-1-84905-027-2 (alk. paper) 1. Cancer--Patients--Great Britain--Biography. 2. Learning disabled--Great Britain--Biography. I. Title.
RC265.5.T84 2010
362.196'9940092--dc22
2009017875

British Library Cataloguing in Publication Data

A CIP catalogue record for this book is available from the British Library

ISBN 978 1 84905 027 2
eISBN 978 0 85700 200 6

This book is dedicated to the
memories of those people whose
stories are told in this book, and
who died between 2005 and 2009

Contents

Acknowledgements

My most heartfelt thanks of all go to the people with learning disabilities who allowed me access to their lives and shared their stories with me. It was a huge privilege to get to know them. I am also deeply grateful to their families and carers, who welcomed me and helped me with my research, sharing their thoughts and feelings with me at a very difficult time. Many of the relatives and carers who were closely involved in the lives of the people in this book took the time to read extracts of the draft of this book. It brought back sometimes painful memories. I am grateful for their generosity in allowing me to publish their stories.

Cancer Research UK generously funded this research and was very supportive throughout the study.

I was extremely fortunate to have many people who supported and encouraged me. I could not have done my research, or written this book, without my colleagues at St George's University of London. Sheila Hollins supervised and guided the study, and pointed me in the right direction when I was stuck. Jane Hubert, an anthropologist whose research experience includes the use of ethnography with people with profound learning disabilities, provided invaluable guidance, not only on how to go about conducting the study but also on how to cope with it. Jane Bernal was always available to talk through my experiences and ideas, and this continued even after she moved to Cornwall. Gary Butler helped me to keep putting myself in the shoes of people with learning disabilities. These colleagues not only listened to me, but also helped me to make sense of my findings. I am particularly indebted to Jane Bernal, whose influence on the analysis is felt throughout the book, and most strongly in the sections about sexuality and about funerals and remembrance.

A research advisory group met regularly throughout the study. I am grateful for the generous support of the following members: Marion MacFarlane and Robert Hill, Service User Development Officers at Merton Learning Disability Services; Catherine Waight, Consultant at Trinity Hospice, Clapham; Adam Penwarden, Director at United Response; Anna Henry, Unit Manager, and Tracy Lazell, Service Manager at the Home Farm Trust; Catherine Farrell, Person Centred Approaches Advisor, and Michaela Gallimore, Practice Development Officer at MacIntyre Care; Carol Boys, Chief Executive, and Susannah Seyman, Information Officer at the Down's Syndrome Association; and Catherine Oakley, Lead Cancer Nurse at St George's Hospital, London. Thank you to Michael Woodman for secretarial support.

The excellent personal supervision and support of Valerie Sinason and Dorothy Judd was invaluable. Without their listening I would have found it too difficult to complete the work.

A number of people read the first draft of this book and gave very helpful feedback on the structure, content and style: Jane Bernal, Leopold Curfs, Lesley Gibbs, Jane Hubert, Sheila Hollins, Astrid Ubas and Astrid Wijne. I am very grateful to them for their considerable time and effort.

Lily Morgan, editor at Jessica Kingsley Publishers, gave me guidance and encouragement during the writing of this book.

Finally, to Michael, Dominic, Clara and Susanna: thank you for your love and patience, and for helping me put life into perspective.

Foreword

Irene Tuffrey-Wijne writes with a passion and freshness that belies the toughness of her research. As her supervisor I can confirm the long hours she spent with people with learning disabilities who were dying, and the close and important relationships she established with so many of the 13 people about whom she writes. She set out to write a book that would be accessible to family members as well as professionals, and does not distract us with the details of her research methods, although these were rigorous and appropriate for the enquiries she wanted to make. This in-depth information is available in academic journals. But her research findings are presented here in the form of readable, detailed accounts of her observations over time as each person's illness progressed and the time of their death approached.

I say readable accounts, but some readers may find parts of these stories distressing. Death and people with learning disabilities has been called 'the last taboo' and it is certainly a subject that has received little airing in academic, professional and policy circles until quite recently. One of the fundamental barriers to open discussion about death is the difficulty we have in finding the right language, emotional vocabulary and understanding within each of our own family and cultural contexts. Communicating with people with learning disabilities about sensitive subjects is no different except that the tools we use to communicate may need to be modified. So for example our listening skills may require patience and confidence on our part as we take note of someone's non-verbal expressions of feeling – not just what he or she says in words. Our explanations and our ability to check how much someone has understood may require us to use non-verbal ways of listening such as prompting him or her with pictures. If we could get it right for people with learning disabilities then we would find talking about death so much easier with other people too!

Irene Tuffrey-Wijne has painstakingly identified common themes that emerged from all of the lives she was privileged to learn about. She has illustrated each theme with excerpts from her field notes, and also reflected on the challenges faced by these 13 people and their carers. There are many learning points for us in these accounts but she has not bombarded us with recommendations, however tempting that might have been! Some of the gaps in service provision, some of the discrimination people seemed to experience and some of the myths about the emotional capacities of people with learning disabilities do point to many obvious areas in which people's last months and days could be better supported. The style of the book leaves readers to draw their own conclusions from their understanding of what is described and explained within it.

The author brings unique skills and experience to her studies, from her dual training as both a palliative care and a learning disability nurse, her experience of working as an assistant in a residential community for people with learning disabilities, and her research training, which resulted in a PhD awarded by the University of Maastricht on this topic.

This book is a good read although not an easy one – I do hope you will be brave enough to read it and share its lessons with your friends, family and professional colleagues.

Sheila Hollins
Professor of Psychiatry of Learning Disabilities,
St George's University of London

Preface

This book describes the lives and illness of 13 people with learning disabilities who had cancer. It looks at their experiences, the care and support they were given, what helped them and what made their lives more difficult. It also looks at the experiences of those around them, their families and paid carers; and it examines the social and health care services that supported them. But first and foremost, this is a book of stories of people with learning disabilities: their own stories, their own perspectives.

I spent three years visiting people at home, at their day centre, in hospital, in a hospice or nursing home. I accompanied them on visits to their GP and came to their hospital outpatient appointments. I sat with them, sharing in their joy, sadness and bewilderment; and I listened to their families, care staff, doctors and nurses. It was a step into the unknown for almost everyone involved, a time full of uncertainty and emotions.

Ten people had died by the time I finished writing this book. Some of these deaths were expected and managed to the best of everyone's ability. Others came as a surprise, despite the cancer: an unexpected phone call that someone had died suddenly. All deaths were a shock, expected or not; an often devastating loss to those left behind. One man was still very ill at the end of my time with him, and was not expected to survive his cancer. There were rays of hope, too. Three people were given the good news that their cancer had gone, although one woman later developed Alzheimer's disease and died of heart failure.

These 13 people were participants in a research study called 'the Veronica Project'. It was named after Veronica Donaghey, a woman with Down's syndrome who had cancer and who wanted her story to be made into a book. She said:

> I'd like the book to be for doctors to read it. A Down's syndrome girl has had cancer twice and pulled through. It's not all bad news. I don't mean doctors are stupid but they are sometimes. I'm not a burden. I help other people. I put something back. It's for everybody really. (Donaghey *et al.* 2002, Introduction)

Veronica's story was turned into a picture book about cancer for people with learning disabilities. Sadly, Veronica died before she could see it in print. Whilst our team at St George's University of London was working on Veronica's book, and evaluating how useful it was for people with learning disabilities, it became clear that we didn't know enough about the experiences of other people with learning disabilities who had cancer, particularly those who were terminally ill. We found, for example, that the carers of some people with learning disabilities would not allow them to read Veronica's book, because they did not want them to know that they had cancer. I wondered about the experiences of these people. I was very fortunate that Cancer Research UK agreed to fund me to spend three years finding out the answers to a very simple question: 'What is it like for people with learning disabilities to have cancer?' A few days after the funding was agreed, I heard about Pete Carpenter, a man with severe learning disabilities who had just been diagnosed with terminal lung cancer. I went to see him and his carers, and he became the first participant in the Veronica Project. Pete died nine weeks later. All 13 people in the Veronica Project had learning disabilities, and they all had cancer. That is where their similarities end. The parameters were set widely. People with learning disabilities are by no means a homogeneous group, and in this study anyone could be included, whether their learning disabilities were mild or profound.

For ease of reference, an overview of the people in this book is given in Appendix 1. All their names are pseudonyms, except those of John Davies and Amanda Cresswell. John and Amanda explicitly asked me to use their real names; the decision to grant their wish was carefully considered by the research advisory group and approved by the research ethics committee (see Appendix 2).

The study included people with all types and stages of cancer: the newly diagnosed, those in remission, and those who were terminally ill. Although the aim was to include people with as wide a variation of cancer experiences as possible, in practice the emphasis was on people for whom a cure was not possible. Somehow, most of the people who were put forward as potential participants were not expected to survive. It was the people who were terminally ill who provided the most poignant data, and as the Veronica Project progressed, it became clear that the focus of the study was gradually shifting from 'having cancer' to 'dying of cancer'. As a result, this book is not only about what it means to have learning disabilities and cancer, but also about what it means to have learning disabilities and die of a progressive illness.

There were three people who were not dying of cancer (Amanda Cresswell, Pauline Deweert and Marion Prentice). Their stories should not, strictly speaking, be part of a book about people who are dying. However, I have included them because these three women provided important insights into the experiences of having learning disabilities and going into hospital, having cancer and coping with treatments. They were also particularly helpful in making me understand ways in which they were resilient. The concepts that emerged from the study were mostly based on the experience of deteriorating health and dying, but the insights provided by Marion, Pauline and Amanda were invaluable.

People with learning disabilities were the focus of the study: they were the ones who were invited to participate, and those around them were in it by default. However, it was inevitable that the families and carers also became study participants, because the experiences of the people with learning disabilities could not be understood in isolation. This book tells their stories, too.

Some of my own story needs to be acknowledged as well. Although it is important that researchers are as objective as possible, in research of this kind they can never leave behind their personal and professional background. This had consequences not only for the kind of information I collected, but also for the way it was interpreted and analysed.

Prior to becoming a researcher, I spent eight years working as a nurse in a hospice, supporting hundreds of terminally ill patients and their families on the wards and in their own homes. I had also spent eight years during the 1980s and 1990s living and working with people with learning disabilities in L'Arche, a vocational community where equal and reciprocal relationships are encouraged. Inevitably this background affected the way I have interpreted and described people's stories. The aim of this book is, of course, to describe *their* stories, not mine; but in this type of research, my own place in these stories and their interpretation cannot be ignored.

My relationship with the people in this book was that of a researcher with study participants. Although I developed warm and close relationships with many of the participants, this professional role was always acknowledged. Most people knew that I was going to write a book about their experiences, and many actively encouraged me in this.

Those who are interested in the methodological details of the study, including ethical issues and details of the analysis, can refer to Appendix 2.

In this book, parts of people's stories are used to explore their experiences, illustrating the themes that have emerged during the study. The demarcation of chapters is somewhat artificial and there are many overlaps. My original field notes are often quoted and printed in italics. For ease of reading, I have set out most speech as quotations, but *these are not always verbatim quotes.* While I have tried to remember people's speech as closely as possible (see Appendix 2), much of it is paraphrased. The only exceptions are parts of John Davies' and Amanda Cresswell's stories, where I used a tape recorder during my first meetings.

The people in this book are by no means representative. There are an estimated 1.2 million people with learning disabilities in England, around 2.5 per cent of the population (Department of Health 2001a). Thirteen people cannot represent this heterogeneous group. The purpose of telling their stories is not to argue that 'this is how it is' for everyone, but to open our eyes to possible feelings, problems and strengths that we may not have considered. My hope is that this will help others to support people with learning disabilities who have cancer, or who are dying, with new insight and understanding. Each person's situation will be different; what we can learn from the people in this book is how individual their needs are and how we can listen better to them. Most of all, I hope that this book will help us see that each person, whether he or she has learning disabilities or not, is important and has a unique story to tell.

CHAPTER 1

Three Stories

This book is a book of stories. Throughout the book, elements of all people's stories will be told to highlight various aspects of their situation. By the end of the book, readers will have a sense of what the people in the Veronica Project went through. Most chapters will begin with part of the story of Lily Lamb, to illustrate the topic of that particular chapter – gradually, her story will be fully told.

However, it is worth telling a few stories from beginning to end. By listening to people's life experiences and following their experiences of illness and dying, I began to appreciate the importance of each person's life and understand some of the impact of what he or she went through. Much understanding can be gained by looking at particular aspects of people's experiences, but some insight comes simply from listening closely to one person and following his or her story from start to finish.

This first chapter tells the stories of John Davies, Vincent Sweeney and Nick Ballard: three men, all with learning disabilities, all with cancer, yet all very different in the way they coped with their life and illness. The other ten stories were important too, and I could have used any of them for this chapter. The experiences of John, Vincent and Nick are not unique in their poignancy, but they will set the scene for the rest of the book.

John Davies

Eight months before he joined the Veronica Project, John Davies was diagnosed with cancer of the penis which had grown to the size of a small melon. It was a shocking diagnosis; even the penile cancer specialists said they'd never seen anything quite like it. However, John had been doing well following the radical surgery that had, so the doctors hoped, removed all the cancer. I first met him on the hospital ward, sitting up in bed, dressed in shorts and a half-open dressing gown. He was keen to meet me, keen to talk – John hardly ever stopped talking, right up to his death nine months later. He was charming and entertaining, with an openness and vulnerability that made it easy for people to like him and to get drawn into his world. He laughed frequently at the memory of good times, but his tears were never far from the surface, ready to flow as he struggled with loss. His dying was saddest of all; he was distressed not so much by losing his life but by losing his beloved family.

John had mild learning disabilities, although this was not immediately obvious and some people doubted it, because he was articulate and had a lovely way with people. Someone John had worked with told me later: 'Learning disabilities, yes, but very mild. He was just one of those people who didn't cope very well with life, who found it difficult.'

That first meeting in hospital came at an anxious time. John's symptoms had returned and he was waiting for the test results. John was captivated by the story of Veronica Donaghey, who had inspired a picture book (Donaghey *et al.* 2002) as well as our research. 'I'm glad she got to tell her story before it was too late,' he said. 'How old was Veronica when she died?' I told him I wasn't sure, but she was probably around 40. 'I am 44,' John pondered. 'I suppose I have done quite a lot in my life, but there are still some things I want to do... Maybe it is a good thing for me to tell my story.'

The following week he was given bad news: the cancer was back. 'The first thing I thought,' he said, 'was, that's it, I am going to make my story into a book. I said to everyone, I'm going to tell my story, warts and all, that's me, everyone can see it.'

From then onwards, John was on a mission. He used the Veronica Project as a way of making sense of his illness and dying, a way of leaving a legacy. He wanted me to bring a tape recorder along so that he could record his story and I could write it down. Sometimes, when I asked him a question, he directed his answer to his imagined audience inside the tape recorder. To his delight we found a journal willing to publish his story, although sadly he died before he could see it in print (Tuffrey-Wijne and Davies 2007). John didn't want to use a pseudonym: 'Sod it, I'm going to use my own name.' It is no coincidence that John's story is the first one in this book, because it was his determination that encouraged me to write it.

John's story in his own words

'Hello, my name is John Anthony Davies, and I am going to tell you my story. I've got cancer, and I don't want to happen to other people what happened to me. I left it far too late.

I was born on the 10 July 1961. I am the eldest son of four brothers. One of my brothers died when he was a baby. His name was Anthony John. My mum is called Margaret.

From the age of one, we discovered that I had a problem with my legs. But the hospital kept saying, "Cut the apron strings, Mrs Davies – there's nothing wrong." They realised too late that there was a problem. I got cerebral palsy in my leg, which is not something that I'd wish on anybody. Name calling is the worst thing that happens, and it's no picnic being called a spastic. But then I've learned to think, "sticks and stones break my bones" and I just kept plodding along, going along in my own little way. But apart from that, I had an amazing childhood. There was lots of love with my mum and my three brothers. My mum raised us the best way she could, always being there when something happened or there was a problem. She was a rock, and is still there, 44 years on. I'm glad to say that I have a wonderful relationship with my mum.

I went to normal schools until I was 14, then I went to a special boarding school for people with learning disabilities. Then tried a few jobs out, working at McDonalds and in a biscuit factory. Then I decided that I wanted to see what the world was like outside. So I walked away from my family for eight long years. They never knew where I was, and I didn't know where they were. Every now and then I'd bump into one of them but I didn't want to know. I wanted to prove that I could live on my own. To say, look, I'm not going to be stuck with you until you're old and grey and I'm collecting pensions for you and me. You know, there is a world out there and I need to go and see it, I need to do things. And if I fall over, then I'll get up and

I'll dust myself off and try again. And if it fails, it fails. It didn't fail. I've been homeless, I slept on the streets, I begged for money when I had no food. It was the silliest thing I've ever done in my entire life, with just a box and no blanket, just the cold.

Life was tough, but then again, in amongst all that was the good bits. I ended up in a hostel, but in the end I walked out of there, not telling them where I was going, and I just walked to a friend's house. My friend and I started singing together in various pubs and clubs. When Paul died, it was the saddest thing that's ever happened. He died of AIDS. He was only 21. I looked after him. And it's very difficult for me to say, that I cannot say I've got a best friend. I *did* have a best friend… Every time I hear "I will Survive", I think of him. That's the song he used to sing. It's been nearly ten years now, but not a day goes by when I don't think of him. I think about the good times we had. And it was him that said, "Look, go and find your mum." Because he never had any contact with his mum…

Anyway, then I decided to see what it would be like working with people who had disabilities like myself, so I started volunteering in respite centres, working with people with disabilities that were worse than my own. I've volunteered with the Orpheus Centre for about 15 years now. We've done all sorts, making music, song and dance, right up my street! I made some wonderful friends along the way. I was privileged to be asked to go to my friend's wedding, and I cried, because I'd never been to a wedding before, not even in my own family. I saw my own friend get married. She looked like a fairy princess.

And all the while I was thinking that one day I would try and find my mum. It's the best thing I've done – I got back in contact with my mum and found out that I've got nieces and a nephew… I keep saying to Paul, I know he can't hear me, but I keep telling him that I found her in the end. And I know he is looking down on me now, and saying, "So you have got cancer. And life will go on." It's him sometimes that makes me feel happy again, like when I used to feel really down and he'd say, "Look, you get like that, let's go and have a drink."

My mum is now not a well woman, but she gets by. When it gets difficult then one of us takes over and helps her out with her shopping and her housework. I like being around my family, knowing that there's somebody to help me out when I need help, and then the same can be said vice versa. So I have a wonderful support network, with my family and my Orpheus friends, although my friends don't come to see me because my family don't like them, they think I've done so much for them and they've done so little for me.

And then I became seriously ill. Quite a while ago I went to the doctor, and I was complaining about a pain when I went to the toilet. The doctor said that it was a urine infection. So they gave me some antibiotics and that was that. Then in August I noticed a lump on my willie, and I just thought it's an infection, the tablets will help it clear up. But it got worse. I just kept thinking it would get better, but all the time it was getting worse. I still did nothing, kept telling myself it would be all right. I never went back to the doctor. I was frightened of what they were going to tell me. And I don't like hospitals at the best of times. I just thought, "No it'll be all right, it'll work itself out." Even when it was really big I still thought it was going to go away. I tried to hide it, because I didn't want people poking their nose in.

I really found it difficult when it got worse. I found it difficult to hide because by then it was noticeable not only to me (I could see it), but everybody else could smell it. There was a bad smell coming, and it didn't matter how many times I got in the bath. One day I got into the bath three times. I got in the bath, got out, dried off, got back into bed, and then it would smell, so I'd get back in the bath. Then if I was going somewhere like my mum's, I would put pads on. I bought Tena Lady pads with stitched-in knickers. I put that on to hide the smell. Then I put two pairs of pants on, so that if the bottom one got wet with a leak I'd have a spare pad and spare knickers to put on. Then I needed to put the belt on as far as I could do it to stop the trousers from falling down. Then I'd walk to the bus stop. Then I'd get out of breath. Then I'd sit on the bus. Then get off that, and get on the train and go round the corner to my mum's house, but before I'd get to the house, I'd put loads of aftershave and deodorant on to stop the smell. But then one day, the smell was that bad, my mum said I hadn't cleaned my bum properly. I remember at Christmas time I was going to my mum's for Christmas dinner, and I didn't want to sit next to anybody because of the smell. I was worried that they would notice it. I worried about the chairs I was sitting on, because of the leaking. I was worried about the chairs getting messy.

And I got really thin. People think I went on a crash diet, which I didn't. You see, some people didn't understand when you have cancer… I didn't know then what I know now, but when you have something serious like that, it doesn't matter how much I was eating. I was still losing the weight because there was something inside killing me.

My mum noticed that I was getting skinny. I said not to worry, that I was OK. But I wasn't really OK at all. And I was very tired. In the end I just went home and went to bed, and I didn't get out for four days. My mum said to my brother, "You go round and see John, I am worried about him." So my brother came round, pretending that he was just passing by and that he wanted a cup of tea. Well, if he wanted a cup of tea he wouldn't have got one because I had the tea bags but no milk: I hadn't been out of bed for four days. I just had bottles of water beside me to drink from, and I was using a bucket to do wee-wee. There was nothing coming out the other end because I weren't eating anything. I'd let it get untidy and there was a bad smell because I couldn't empty the bucket that had the wee-wee in. I hadn't been able to keep the house clean, everything that was in the house smelled of wee-wee. Later on the council had to come and fumigate the whole house. When my brother came he just took one look at me. I tied the coat round me but the coat fell off and he saw this lump, and this stuff coming out of it… It made him feel sick. He just got on the phone and called the ambulance there and then. And I got carted off to hospital.

I can't cope with the fact that my brother saw the way that I was when I was taken into hospital. It's just something that's stuck in his head. I have watched him. He was crying, and said, "Mum, I can't describe what I saw that day. It's in my head when I go to bed and it's in my head when I wake up." He'll never forget it, and I wish there was something that I could do to alleviate the pain that he must be going through. My family have all said that they would take my pain away if they could, and they would all have my illness, but I wouldn't wish my illness on anybody. But I am glad that my brother came. The doctors said that if he hadn't gone and sent me into hospital, I would be dead now. So really I am grateful to my mum for sending my brother round.

A doctor told me that I'd got cancer, and at first you think, oh dear, cancer – that's a terrible word. I got diagnosed in March with penile cancer, and then in April I had the whole lot taken away from me. My bits and pieces, my bladder and my bowel, everything. They didn't know if I was going to live or die. I often think that I'm going to beat it. The doctors said that they had taken all the cancer away. Now I take one day at a time. Life is too short, so I take one day at a time. You try to make the best out of a bad thing, which is what I have been trying to do.

I think the worst bit that came out of all of this was having to tell my mum that I'd got cancer. At first I thought I wouldn't tell people, but then I just braced myself and said to everybody that I know, "I've got cancer." I know it is a terrible word, but you've got to get used to it. And they cried, and I cried… I cried enough tears to fill a river. But then I said, "Look, don't cry any more, go and have a cry somewhere else. Then come back, give me a cuddle and tell me how you've been, and what's going on in the world, because that's what I need to know. Tell me something nice."

We carried along, and I got better again. The bandages came off, and because there had been so much surgery on my legs, I had to start walking again, so with the help of physiotherapy I managed to walk. They got me somewhere to live, and they were going to let me out of hospital, but it wasn't ready for moving into because it had to be adapted. I couldn't go back to my old flat because that had stairs in it, and they wanted somewhere for me to have no stairs, so they found me a ground floor flat. I had to wait a bit for it, and they wanted the hospital bed, so they shoved me in a residential care home, an old folks home – I was the youngest person in the room. Living in my own flat didn't work out. I lived miles away from my family and it got lonely. The carer would come in and do the housework, and stick me in the bath, the district nurse would come and do the dressing, but if it was raining it got so lonely. I couldn't go anywhere, and if nobody came to visit me, I sat watching the TV or watching the same DVDs over and over again. At one point I could sit there and sing every song from Sister Act I and II with Whoopi Goldberg in. And I would phone people up, saying, "Here I am, I'm all right Jack, blah, blah, blah…" It's better being with my mum. I'm living with her now. She wants me to, and I worry sometimes that it is too much for her, but I know that she would worry more about me if I lived somewhere by myself.

Things were OK for a while, but then it all started to leak again, and I had to go back to hospital. They did some more tests. Then came the bad news: the cancer had come back. It was awful. The worst of it was telling my mum. She was so upset. I cried as well, we all cried. I really thought the cancer had gone, but they said that a little bit has come back. They said they were going to give me chemotherapy to get rid of that little bit. They let me go home for Christmas and then started the chemo in January.

Since then I have been in hospital a couple of times. Once I got really sick, I was vomiting in the street. I could see the people in the bus looking at me and laughing, they probably thought I was drunk. And I got terrible diarrhoea and stomach pains and fevers. So they sorted me out in hospital and then I could go home again. The pains are still quite bad sometimes. I am taking morphine now. I don't think there's much more they can do for me. They said that if the chemo doesn't work it's going to kill me, and it isn't working, so... I've resigned myself to the fact that I'm going to be in and out of hospital, in, out, up and down, up and down, like a stripper's knickers!

It can be hard. Sometimes I sit in the hospital bed feeling miserable, and I think, "Right, in the next ten minutes they'll all turn up to visit me," so I take a deep breath, put a smile on, and I sit there for half an hour or so talking about silly things. I've done that plenty of times, make out that I'm all right when inside I'm not, I'm just fed up.

I don't know how long I've got left...and I want to do so many things, and tell so many people things before I get taken away. I just can't stop telling my mum how much I love her, because I'm going to miss my mum, and it's going to be a terrible wrench. I am not ready to go yet. There are things I want to do in my life. But I hope it's quick if it comes. I hope it is in my sleep. And I want it to be at home with my mum. I do think about where it is going to happen. I worry about my mum. They don't want me to die in pain. That's what I don't want: having them see me in terrible pain. But the doctors and nurses have said that I don't have to die in pain. I want to go in my sleep.

But apart from that, I'm all right... It's no good moaning. There's a whole world out there, so much to do and to see, what should I be sitting here for feeling sorry for myself? You need to make the best of it. I say a prayer every evening and I say a little prayer every morning, thankful for having been given another day. Every day is another day with my family. We may not do much, just sitting here watching the telly, but that's what is important, just being together, spending time together.

So this is my story. This is a real story that comes from the heart. I did not make any of it up. What I want to say to you is this:

> Look, if you notice anything different to how it was before, then for God's sake, go and see someone! I left mine too late, but you need to go to the doctor. The two things I don't like in life are going to the doctor, and going to the dentist. But for God's sake, you've got to go and see somebody and say, "Look… It's only small." Mine was small – but then mine got big. Believe me, you do not want to go through what I've gone through. I have sat there and watched my family suffer tremendously. Sometimes I think: I wish… But you could wish a thousand wishes, and there is nobody with a magic wand to make it better. Sometimes I look at myself and think, I lost my dingly-danglies. And I could have saved them. And now I've lost the chance of any kind of relationship with anybody.

If there's a way of this story helping somebody else, if it can help somebody to possibly save themselves from all the stuff that me and my family have been through, then I'll be happy. I think I was put on Planet Earth to help people. So if my story can stop someone from getting cancer, who knows… If that helps, then I am ever blessed.'

Final months

This is where John ended the story he told his imagined audience, in May 2006 – but it is not the end of his story. He deteriorated gradually, slowly losing energy and the ability to walk. Sometimes he lost concentration, staring into space before bringing himself back with a jolt. The surgery wounds in his groin began to sprout odorous cancer nodules, and sometimes he found that there was a sudden flood of blood pouring down his legs. He dealt with this in a matter-of-fact way, as if it was just one of life's many chores. His deterioration was almost imperceptible, because he steered his focus away from his increasing limitations and pain, away from himself and onto others. 'Oh,

I'm all right, how are *you*?' he said to his visitors. When it became clear the chemotherapy was not helping him, he accepted his fate but he was distraught for his family's sake. 'I'm relieved that I don't have to have the treatments any more, but I'm disappointed too, because I can't give any more comfort to my mum.'

John no longer wanted to talk into a tape recorder. He had talked a lot about his desire to record a CD for his funeral, and had clear plans for what he was going to say: 'Hello! Ta-ra! Here I am, you thought you'd be rid of me but I'm not quite gone yet, I'm still here. And I love you all.' I offered to help and left him the recording equipment, but it was just too difficult. He could never get the words out without crying.

In July, John's mother was suddenly taken into intensive care. She was suffering from respiratory failure, and for a few weeks it was uncertain whether she would survive. John's brothers tried to combine visiting her in hospital with looking after John, who by now needed a considerable amount of physical care, but it was too much. John went into a hospice for respite care. He realised immediately that he needed a new plan for the future. 'Me and my brother have been talking about it. The others say, "Don't be daft, it'll be all right." But we say, "What if it isn't?" I know I have to be realistic. She may not come home. And if she does come home, she cannot look after me. And I can't look after myself. So I will need to find somewhere else to live. She won't like it, and she will say that she is OK, but I will have to tell her, "Mum, your days of looking after me are done." I am very ill, and she can't look after me. So I think they are going to look for some sort of home for me, because I can't stay here forever either.'

Three weeks later, he moved into a nursing home. He was happy to be there, happy not to have to worry about burdening his family any more. He had his own room with his own TV and music. He quickly made friends and he threw himself into the weekly karaoke sessions.

However, not everything in the nursing home was ideal. I spoke to the manager about the fact that they had pinned John's care plan up on his wardrobe door, plain for all to see, containing sensitive and confidential information about him and his family. Some aspects of the home upset John too. He described the lady who served him breakfast: 'She was talking about me, like "What can he eat?" and

"What does he like?", just as if I wasn't there. I didn't like that at all. It really upset me, I was crying. "Don't treat me like that," I said. "I am here, you can talk to me."'

John was worried about his mother, but he turned his mind to something positive. The hospice created the opportunity for him to go on stage in a local theatre, complete with a musician and a group of young dancers, so that he could record something for his family. This work continued when he was in the nursing home; he kept attending the hospice day centre every week. John planned his performance in detail and rehearsed for weeks before recording a DVD with a song and a message of love for his mother. The last time I spent with John, he had just received the DVD in the post. He watched it with tears in his eyes, and I couldn't help crying with him. He wanted to be reassured that his story would be published under his own name. 'Now I've achieved everything,' he told me. I didn't realise the significance of his words until later. 'Some friends of mine had something wrong with them, and I told them to go and see a doctor. I said to them, "Look where I am, I didn't go to the doctor, and now I'm on my way to heaven."' He looked at me and added, 'Because I am, you know. On my way to heaven.'

John died suddenly two days later.

Dying and beyond

The hospice nurse, who visited the nursing home to support John and to advise the nurses, told me what had happened. 'I saw him the day before he died. It was pain problems, mainly. I think he was in an awful lot of pain. I increased his morphine. But the nurses said they were really struggling with his pain and his wound. They said that his wound had completely broken down, and his internal organs were almost on view. The next day he had woken up in the morning. He struggled to take his medicine, which is when the nurses rang me again. I packed my emergency kit and was on my way, but by the time I arrived he had already died. He had asked for a bit of breakfast, and the nurses started giving him some. The nurses were lovely. But then one of the nurses realised that he was actually dying. They just sat with him. He died quickly, within an hour.'

John's death was a huge shock to his family. His mother was back home by now, being looked after by two of her sons. John had managed to visit her a few weeks earlier. His youngest brother told me of their anger and distress at what happened when John died.

'I'd gone to the home in the evening to watch Eastenders with him. Just to keep him company. I said to the bloke on Reception that I was going up to see John, and he went all funny. He said, "Hold on a minute" and phoned someone. He was mumbling in the phone like this, and I got a funny feeling then. Then he said, "If you go upstairs someone will be waiting for you," so I went up and there was one of the nurses. Offering me a cup of tea. They told me he had died 12 hours ago.'

The nursing home staff said that they tried to phone the family but didn't have the right number. It seemed rather extraordinary that this was so. John had been at the nursing home for five weeks; during that time he had talked about his mother and brothers every day, and his family had visited him frequently. John's brother, deeply shocked, asked to see John, but John's body had already been taken away. His brother demanded to know where, but the nurses didn't know the details. 'I lost it then,' John's brother said. 'I completely freaked out, I was shouting at them, and they phoned the police. That was the final straw. I said to the police, "Look, I have just found out that my brother has been dead for 12 hours, that he is in a fridge somewhere and nobody can tell me where, and now I've got to go home and tell my mum that her son is dead. That's her second son who has died. Can you see where I am coming from?!" And he just looked at me, this big burly policeman, and he said, "Yes, I can actually."'

John's mother was utterly devastated by his death. 'How can I celebrate Christmas if my heart has been broken and it can't ever be mended?' she cried. 'It is like a big hole in my heart, and I don't think it can ever be filled. He is my first-born. He was always with me when he was a boy, always, wherever I went. Of all my boys, he was the one who always stayed close. When I went out, shopping or whatever, he would always come. He would ask, "Where are you going, Mum?" And I'd say, "Out of my mind." And he would ask, "Can *I* come?" I just cannot believe that I will never see him again.' John's mother died seven months later, and there was no doubt in the mourners' minds that with John's death she had lost the will to live.

John's brothers carried his coffin into the crematorium. One brother read out the poem John had so much wanted to record in his own voice for this very occasion. The minister painted a picture of a man who was lovely and friendly but who didn't have an easy life. 'Of course, he was born with a disability, but he never let it stop him from having a positive attitude. He was always singing, from when he was very young…whatever life threw at him, he just kept on singing.'

Later, I watched John's DVD many times, and never stopped being moved by him singing 'If happy little bluebirds fly beyond the rainbow, Mum, oh why can't I?'

Vincent Sweeney

Vincent Sweeney was 47 years old and lived on his own. He had been diagnosed with lung cancer, and I was told by the palliative care nurse who put his name forward for the Veronica Project that he was very keen to join. He needed someone to listen to him. I met with Vincent regularly for two years, and I could not have predicted how much I would learn from him.

Vincent welcomed me into his flat with flair, making tea for me and his sister-in-law. He had excellent social skills, with an easy chat and a ready smile, and as with John, his mild learning disabilities weren't immediately obvious when you first met him. He was a large man, with neatly combed grey hair and an oversized stomach. But despite his initially cheery exterior, there were times when his low mood made him grumpy and unapproachable, and it didn't usually take him long to start talking about the things that were missing in his life. Support from outside agencies. People to sort out his life for him. Friends. Vincent was deeply lonely. He had spent most of his adult life living in hostels and foster care, within services for drug and alcohol addiction rather than for learning disabilities. He had 'messed up' these placements more than once, unable to stay because of his sometimes volatile or violent behaviour. He regretted this, blaming the drink.

Vincent moved into his own flat two years ago. He liked the new independence it gave him, the sense of being in control, and he was rightly proud of his achievements, particularly in saving money. 'Now

I've got money to go out and do what I like!' he said, and he was careful not to lose it. He gave all his money for safe keeping to Susan, his sister-in-law, because he knew he would otherwise spend it on drink and gambling. He could not have imagined that this money would later pay for his funeral.

Susan and Donald (Vincent's older brother) lived nearby and were his main support. Susan telephoned him every day, and he visited her every Tuesday. On a Sunday he could turn up at their house and they would give him lunch. She scolded him for his bare cupboards, for not eating healthily, surviving on beans on toast for breakfast, lunch and supper, supplemented by take-away chips.

Vincent had a part-time job with the local council, working at the reception desk where he would answer the telephone. He worked five days per week, for just an hour at 7am and again at 7pm, but he would hang around in between, chatting to people and having lunch with his colleagues. He had been in the job for ten years and he loved it. It got him out of the house. It gave his day structure, leaving early in the morning and returning well into the evening. Then the day would be almost over and he wouldn't have to face his loneliness.

A few professionals were important in his life, people he looked to for ongoing support. The learning disability nurse; his counsellor; his social worker. Later, this inner circle of professionals also included his palliative care nurse and myself. What he really craved was their friendship and total commitment, the assurance that he wasn't alone in life, but in this he was invariably disappointed.

Childhood

Vincent grew up in London, the fourth of five children born to Irish parents. He attended a mainstream school but couldn't keep up. Other children called him 'dumb'. 'That hurt,' he said. At his teachers' advice, his parents sent him to a far-away boarding school for children with special needs. Vincent remembered how the strict nuns would get the slipper out when you misbehaved, and how he yearned to go back home with his parents whenever they visited. When he went home for holidays, the children in the neighbourhood teased him: 'You're dim, you're going to a special school.' Vincent never learned to read or write properly; when presented with written text, he just picked out the easiest words and skipped the rest. Even now he sometimes misunderstood what a newspaper story was about.

Susan described Vincent's longing for friendships. 'I don't think Vincent has *any* friends. Never had. Not really. He wants to. He will *buy* his friends. He'll buy everyone a round in the pub, but then when he has no money, no one will buy him one back. Even when he lived with his mum and dad, he would buy people presents, hoping that they would be his friends, but he never really got friends.'

Vincent himself said: 'When the school finished I wanted to be part of a gang. And they were all drinking and smoking. So I did too, and I got into trouble. I knocked down a man. I just wanted to be part of a gang and everything like that.'

This beginning of a lifelong struggle with drink and violence, and a deep desire to belong, coincided with a painful experience of being sexually abused. It left him traumatised, to the extent that even now, some 30 years later, he felt unable to sustain – or even start – a loving relationship. Anyway, he sighed, it was too late for him to start a relationship now that he was grey and ill. He had missed his chance. 'I would really like a girlfriend,' he said. 'What I want is to have someone who understands, someone to go out with, for a meal or to the cinema. I don't want to go down the pub all the time. But I can't have a relationship. That was well and truly effed up. I look at my brothers and sister, Steven is married with kids, Donald is married with kids, Sinead's got kids, Kevin does, and I… I have nothing.'

Vincent's happiest childhood memories involved spending time with his father, whom he adored. 'I was close to my dad. He worked, he went out in the morning and didn't come home until late at night and demand a dinner, and my mum would already be in bed. But on a Sunday after the 10 o'clock mass he would take me down the pub with him, and he would down a few pints… And when he worked I would go out and meet him. I could see all the vans going past: white van, no, that's not him; another white van, that's not him either; a red van, a blue van, that's not him; a white van…there he is! And we would go home together. He'd say, "How was your day?" and I'd say, "OK." "How's mum?" "She's fine. She is getting the dinner ready." I miss my dad. I still miss him sometimes.'

When Vincent was in his twenties and the only one of the siblings still living at home, his parents moved back to Ireland. His father died 15 years ago. Vincent went to the funeral. He spoke repeatedly of his desire to go back to Ireland to see his father's grave, to talk to his father, and the gradual realisation that this would not be possible for him – he was too tired and too frightened of the journey – was painful. At one point I asked him whether he might be able to talk to his father here, at home. What would he say?

> *He says immediately: 'Hello dad, I miss you. I've got cancer. The family is all right. They're looking after me.' Vincent adds, talking to me now, 'I do talk to him, you know. Sometimes at night, I speak to him. People say I'm mad, that he is dead, he has died, he's gone, I should leave it behind and move on. The past is past. But I can't. I sometimes feel he is still here.'*
>
> *I tell Vincent that he is not mad. 'Vincent, people that you have loved like that, and who have loved you like your father loved you, they are never going to go away. They are always part of you, and they are always here.' He says: 'Yes, and I could always talk to my dad… I would go to him with my problems and say, "Dad, can I talk to you?"'*
>
> *I say, 'Vincent, you really have problems now. If you told them to your dad now, what would he say to you?' Again, Vincent doesn't have to think about this. He says, 'Get on with your life, son. I'm here, I'm always here, and you just get on with your life.'*
>
> *Vincent just stares ahead of him. His face is tense, and I feel he is in a different world where he is completely and utterly present with his father. When he comes back to me he says, 'You know, my life changed when my mum and dad went back to Ireland. I miss that. I miss my old life. I miss my life with them.'*

Cancer

When Vincent started complaining of not feeling well (shortness of breath, coughing up blood, weight loss), his family had their doubts. Susan explained, 'We didn't believe him at first when he became ill. Because he likes to be ill. Always has done. He used to make up illnesses, he was at the GP and Accident and Emergency all the time with pain in his chest and things like that, and they could never find anything wrong with him. So when he really was ill, we didn't believe him at first. Not until the doctor said.'

Just before Christmas, Vincent was diagnosed with lung cancer. He had vivid memories of being told that he had cancer. 'It was such a shock when they told me. The doctor said, "I have some bad news for you." So I said, "Hold on, don't tell me now, I need my family with me." So I called them and they came. They were around the bed, Susan and Donald, Steven, Sinead. The doctor said: "There is no nice way of saying this, Vincent. You've got cancer." I couldn't take it. I had to go out, I smoked three cigarettes in five minutes, and I was crying and crying. Later, I saw out of the corner of my eye that Susan was crying when she left. I have never seen her cry before. That was really upsetting... They said I'd be dead by next Christmas.'

Vincent was given chemotherapy, but that was stopped because it had no effect. Radiotherapy might have been more effective and this was started, but Vincent did not see it through, being somewhat scared of the radiotherapy machine. He was now simply monitored at the hospital outpatients clinic, which he attended every three months for an X-ray and a talk with the doctor.

He was also referred to the local palliative care team based at the hospice. He started attending the hospice day centre, which he enjoyed enormously. It took him out of the house. 'I love it at the centre,' he said. 'The time flies by. Everyone is so friendly there. It is like a family. I like company. I like having people to talk to. I used to go to work all day and talk to my colleagues, but now I can't. And I had a really good learning disabilities team. I had the same nurse for 15 years. I still used to go and see them sometimes. I'd get up early and go on the bus, and when I came back it was 8 o'clock, have a bit of supper, and it's time for bed. Great. Another day finished... But I can't do that any more. I get too tired, and then I get aggressive.'

Pain, loneliness, fear and distress

Vincent's constant complaints of pain exasperated his family and professionals alike. The first thing I was told about him, both by his hospice nurse and by Susan and his sister Sinead, was that he told everyone a different story about his pain, making it very difficult to know how to help him. Sometimes he would ring Sinead, crying desperately, leaving a message on her mobile to say that he was having terrible pains. Sinead, who lived too far away to drop in, would then ring Donald and Susan to check, only to find that Vincent was with them and that he seemed fine.

Although I never doubted the reality of Vincent's pain – he took a fairly high dose of morphine for it – what he told me about it made it clear that fear and anxiety were at the root of his pain problems, and that this would make it difficult or even impossible to control with medication alone. 'I get really lonely here,' he explained a few weeks after I first met him. 'I worry or I panic. Sometimes I sit here and there is something on TV that makes me panic, like when they talk about cancer. Then I ring people up, and they ask me what's wrong, so I tell them that I am having pain. I'm not in pain really, I am just lonely and worried. But I can't keep ringing people up, can I? I can't keep ringing Susan every five minutes just because I am lonely. She has her own life to live.'

Complaints of pain and of not being able to sleep were usually the first thing he told me when I visited, and it was only after I had listened intently for a few minutes without offering any suggestions that he would move on to telling me about his fears and loneliness. After a year of this it was easy to see how hard it could be for the people around him. The number of tablets he had to take each day ran into double figures, and although the district nurses organised them for him, he was sometimes confused about the extra morphine he could take. Four months after we met, he admitted to me that he often threw all his tablets in the bin, although he realised he needed his morphine and still took that most days.

What caused him the most worry was thinking about his cancer and all the things he had been told by doctors and nurses. What did it all mean? He wanted answers, but any answers he was given sent him into bleak depths of fear. The things he had been told would go round and round in his head; he mulled over any suggestions of further investigations or treatments again and again. 'I get pains. The GP sent me for an X-ray of my back. I don't know why. I lie awake at night worrying about it. I've got no one to talk to. I can't sleep. I don't know what the X-ray is for. Are they trying to see if the cancer has spread?'

Vincent wanted as many professionals as possible to support him, but couldn't cope with their different approaches and different suggestions. When the doctor from the hospice day centre gave him anti-depressants, he poured out his confusion. 'One doctor says that I am OK, that I can go back to work if I am feeling 100 per cent. Then there is my doctor [GP] who says that I should go and have a holiday whilst I still can. What is that supposed to mean? Whilst I still can? And now the hospice doctor says I need stress tablets. I don't know who to believe. It is going round and round in my head, and I don't know what to think. So I go into my bedroom and I shut the door, and I just cry. That's what I do. Because I am upset and I don't know what is going on. And then I look at my father's photograph.'

Vincent was looking for people to support him, but no one could live up to his expectations. 'I'm not getting the help I need' was a frequent refrain. People who did genuinely try to help him (his social worker, his hospice nurse) would eventually fall out of favour, because nobody was able to sort out his deep-seated problems. He fluctuated easily between singing people's praises and cursing them. One by one, the trusted professionals fell away, leaving their job or discharging him from their caseload. His hospice nurse passed on her responsibilities to the day centre staff. She had been at a complete loss about his pain control, and maybe did not quite appreciate how much her listening ear meant to Vincent. Anyway, his trust in her had taken a serious dent when he discovered that she had told Susan about his complaints and demands. What he talked about with his nurses, he fumed, ought to be confidential.

Understanding cancer

Much of Vincent's anxiety was around his understanding, or lack of understanding, of cancer and what was happening to him. His tendency to mull things over was almost unbearable when it came to his panics about the meaning of cancer, keeping him awake for weeks, sometimes months.

'I had an X-ray last week, and then talked to the doctor about it,' he complained. 'I don't know what happened. He had the picture up on the screen, and he said, "It looks all right but I want a second opinion." I can't understand that. What does he want to have a second opinion for if it looks all right? We wanted to find out if the cancer had spread, but he didn't say anything about that. All he said was that he wants a second opinion and that it looks all right. I can't understand things like that. The doctor talks to me and I can't understand it. I have learning disabilities, I don't understand talk like that. Susan understands, and Sinead, so they talk to the doctor. They can put it much better than I can. All I want to do is get away from the doctor's room and go out and have a fag, but I am stuck, because Susan and Sinead are sitting between me and the door. So I have to stay.'

I accompanied him on his next outpatients appointment. The experience of not being heard and not understanding left Vincent furious; he was going to report that doctor, kill him even: only the presence of Susan and myself had stopped him from such a crime, he said.

> *The doctor fires a few questions. 'Any pain?' 'Yes, here,' says Vincent (indicating his liver area). 'Do you get breathless?' Vincent doesn't quite know what the doctor means. His hesitation prompts the doctor to qualify, 'How far can you walk on the flat?' 'I'm OK,' says Vincent. 'I'm not good with hills. I get out of breath then.' 'Would you have breathing problems if you were sitting still?' 'I'd rather keep active,' says Vincent. He clearly has no clue what this questioning is all about. The doctor peppers his talk with words like 'instigate treatment' and 'correlate how you are feeling with the X-ray results'. They are not on the same wavelength. They speak different languages.*

Reflecting on this appointment afterwards, Vincent was very clear what he wanted to know from the doctor. Susan and the palliative care nurse pointed out to me later that these were questions he often asked, but I felt that he either had not been given clear answers, or he had not taken them on board. 'What is happening with the cancer?' Vincent started his list of questions. 'Has it shrunk or is it spreading? I know it hasn't gone. Or at least I don't think it has! I don't think cancer just goes away. But is the cancer getting smaller or is it growing? And where exactly is it in my body? Are they going to give me any more treatment for it? Or are the doctors even just *thinking* about giving me more treatment? I don't mind them telling me that they don't know. But they should just tell me. I want to know... What is the cause of my pains? Why can't I sleep? What caused the cancer? Is it the drink? Is it the smoke? I am smoking more now.'

I offered to help him ask these questions at his next appointment. Vincent was extremely nervous beforehand, but this time his experience with the same doctor was completely different. The doctor's information was no different from before: the X-rays showed no growth in the cancer, and further treatment would only be given if symptoms occurred; the aim of such treatment would be comfort, not cure. But with my help the doctor answered all Vincent's questions in simple words and carefully explained everything we could see on the X-ray. Afterwards Vincent didn't feel angry and confused, but elated. The only time the doctor reverted to more difficult medical language was when Vincent asked him, 'There is nothing to worry about then, is there. Is it life-threatening? It isn't going to kill me or anything?'

The doctor exchanges glances with Susan and Sinead. I can't see what the looks on their faces are, because I am watching Vincent and the doctor. The doctor hesitates slightly before giving his answer: 'At some time in the future, the tumour may well progress. But at the moment, things are OK. So there is nothing to worry about for the moment. It is only when you become symptomatic that we would worry.' The sisters are quick to agree: 'Yes, so there is nothing to worry about right now.' At this stage, Vincent is smiling.

Vincent was aware of the fact that he found it hard to live with the uncertainties of cancer. He wanted to know everything people said about him, and yet he didn't.

'I think Susan and Sinead know things that I don't know. They aren't telling me. They keep it from me, because they think I couldn't cope.'

Are they right? Could he not cope with knowledge about his cancer? He agrees with them. He doesn't think he could. 'When they told me I had cancer, I just lost it,' he says. 'I couldn't cope with it.' 'But you cannot cope now either,' I point out. 'You are sitting here, or lying in your bed, and you don't know or understand what is going on, and it is hard for you.' He agrees with that too. I ask him, 'Are you frightened?' 'Yes,' he says. 'I'm scared.'

Family

Vincent continued to visit his colleagues every week, taking the bus to travel to the work place. Gradually, it became obvious that he wouldn't be able to return to his job. Although he had good days, he couldn't be relied upon because he was often too tired. Vincent kept up hope, and it was a great blow when he was told that his job had been given to someone else. Colleagues who initially kept in regular contact began to fade away.

The hospice day centre compensated in some way for this loss. Vincent enjoyed the company of other patients, the sharing of common experiences. It could be hard, though, that the people he had friendly chats with one day would not be there the next, and he would find out that they had died. He made friends with Frank. They were two lonely friends who needed each other, telephoning each other frequently. Frank's death hit Vincent hard.

Throughout it all, Vincent's family kept him going. He often exasperated them, annoying them, even infuriating them with his inconsistent complaints. Susan fumed, 'He is lying. He is telling each person a different lie. He lied to me for weeks. He told me he had the scan when he hadn't, and only came clean a few weeks later. And I went with him! I sat outside in the corridor when he came out and said that he'd had the scan! I suppose he had to tell me in the end, because when we go to his appointment tomorrow to get the results, there won't be any results because he never had the scan. Twice I went with him. I make a big effort, I have a job and need to take time off, and then he doesn't have it and bloody lies to me about it.'

Vincent was distressed by her anger, anxious that Susan might abandon him, conscious of how badly he had treated her. But she never abandoned him, and neither did the rest of his family. They were deeply committed, and Vincent knew this. He sang their praises almost every time I visited.

Vincent yearned for his mother, yet could not reach her. Vincent spoke to her on the phone every fortnight, but he usually pretended that he was OK. 'I lie,' he said. 'I lie to my mum. She asks, "How are you?" and I say, "I'm fine." I can't tell her, she would only worry. She's 84. I can't talk to her about how I'm not feeling well. My family won't let me. They say I have to tell her I'm fine.'

His mother came over from Ireland occasionally, staying with Susan and Donald, but Vincent said he did not know what to say to her then. Despite his longing he would often ignore her. He did the same with his sister Sinead, whom he would sometimes ring up, imploring her to come, yet when she did he acted as if she wasn't there. It puzzled and frustrated his family. Vincent's family was often on his mind, he needed them, he worried about them, but he was unable to express this to them. Once, when he complained about doctors just giving him tablets to help him sleep (what good were more tablets going to do him?), I asked him.

> *'What is it, Vincent? What is it that keeps you awake? What are you worrying about?' He answers with his usual readiness: 'My family. My mother. Whether I'm going to be able to go back to work or not.' I ask, 'Tell me more. What is it that worries you about your family?' He looks at me... And for the first time during our meetings, he stops sitting on the edge of the seat, he stops fidgeting. He leans back into the sofa, he rests his head, and his eyes fill with tears as he looks at me. For the first time, it is as if the ever present armour has come off, the ever present sense that he could fly into a rage at any moment, that he could suddenly pull down the shutters and raise his fists to protect himself, physically and emotionally...*
>
> *'I miss my mum. She was here last month and I want to see her. I want to go and see my father's grave. But I don't think I am going to be able to get there. I can't fly for two hours. And I can't tell my mum everything. She can't take it. I worry about Donald. And Susan. I love them more than anything, they mean the world to me. They are always there for me. And I treat Susan like dirt. I want to be with my family...'*
>
> *He snaps out of this vulnerable state, sits up, curses the awful doctor once more, although he always consciously minds his language in my presence.*

Vincent worried about the future. What made life difficult was the fact that the things that had kept him going in the past – his job, his trips out of the house, to the shops or the pub – were slowly eroded by his illness. After losing his job he also gradually became too tired and short of breath just walking outside, and it meant that he was looking at the four walls of his flat for most of the day. It was a conundrum that was obvious to most people, yet no one knew how to solve it. Vincent was just about coping at the moment, supported by Susan and by home helps who cleaned and shopped for him twice a week, but nobody voiced the unspoken worry: what will happen when Vincent becomes too ill to cope at home? As it turned out, the question never needed answering.

Death

Vincent died suddenly and unexpectedly, exactly two years after my first meeting with him. When I telephoned him the week before he had sounded his usual self: 'I still can't sleep, I'm not getting the help I need, what's the point of going to see the doctor, all they do is talk talk talk, why don't they tell me what's happening with the cancer, has it grown, has it shrunk, why can't they sort out the pain?' At an outpatients appointment that week, Vincent was told that he was doing well; in fact, the cancer looked no bigger on the X-ray.

Susan told me what happened next. 'He didn't turn up at the hospice day centre on the Monday, so they rang me and I went round to see him. My son was with me. I think the cancer had burst. There was blood absolutely everywhere. The kitchen was full of blood, and he had taken all his clothes off. We found him naked in his bedroom. He must have taken off his clothes to try and wipe up the blood, because his clothes were on the kitchen floor as if he'd tried to wipe it. His bedroom was also full of blood. He was on the phone when he died, I don't know who he was trying to ring, an ambulance or me. My son had such a shock, he is in quite a state, still is. They said in the hospice that the cancer must have burst a blood vessel. And that he probably died quickly, no more than a couple of minutes… It was awful.' Susan continues: 'We think it must have happened on the Sunday afternoon or early evening. His brother rang him on the Sunday at 12 o'clock, and he said he wasn't feeling very well. But Vincent always said he wasn't feeling very well, so we didn't really think much of it. When I found him, his television page was still on the Sunday. And all his Sunday evening tablets were still there. I know he didn't always take them, but still. And I don't think it happened in the evening or at night, because none of the lights were on. Vincent would always have put the lights on. He was scared of the dark.'

It is, thankfully, fairly unusual for a cancer patient to bleed to death the way Vincent did. Vincent may or may not have realised the implications of vomiting so much blood, but he was clearly conscious for long enough to take action, trying to clean up the blood, trying to phone for help. Nobody could have prevented Vincent dying the way he did, but the manner of his death was terribly sad, because it reflected so poignantly the way he had lived: alone and lonely, very frightened, and – in his own, often repeated words – 'not getting the help'.

Nick Ballard

The situation of Nicholas Ballard, or Nick as he was usually called, was very different from John's and Vincent's. Nick had Down's syndrome and severe learning disabilities, and needed much support in life. Nick could not tell me his story in words, and in order to find out what his life was like I spent many hours with him over a period of nine months. I talked a lot with the people who supported him, in particular his home manager Mary – this is her story, too. My focus was always on Nick and I did my best to look at the world through his eyes, but the interpretation of what I saw, and of his communication and behaviour, are more strongly my own than in the previous two stories.

Nick was 56 years old, but his deeply lined face looked older. His small head had only a few wisps of grey hair that had once been dark. He had big brown eyes with which he gazed intently at people and things that interested him. He was slightly stooped and had the walk of a man full of purpose who knows what he wants. Nick did not speak and was severely deaf. He communicated by making sounds and using Makaton signs,[1] although staff at his day centre and his residential care home only used basic Makaton vocabulary. The day centre staff did not know the sign for 'pain'. Nick did.

Nick liked things to be tidy and organised. Tables had to be cleared, chairs pushed straight, and people should be where they belonged, doing what they ought to do. He wiped splashes off tables and paint off his fingers, sometimes onto someone else's sleeve. He tidied coffee cups away even before people had finished, much to the annoyance of his peers at the day centre and the bemusement of his fellow patients in hospital. He was sublimely self-centred, ordering people to move out of his way in a manner that tolerated no resistance if they happened to sit at a lunchtime table that he had earmarked for himself. He was very clear about who 'his' support workers were and would greet them with a heart-melting smile and a hug, then demand that they stay at his side. He could be rude to other people with learning disabilities, gesturing full of disapproval or pushing them if he didn't like what they did. He had been on medication for his behaviour for more years than anyone remembered. Mary, his home manager, was unsure why the medication had been started, but sometimes wondered whether he had serious mental health problems, maybe even hallucinations.

Despite being described by his carers as strong-willed, Nick was clearly used to being told what to do. He often followed instructions meekly and without questioning: 'Take your jumper off,' 'Don't do that.' Once he got used to hospital routines, he obliged without question when nurses took blood or asked him to lie down.

Nick loved sports, waving flags enthusiastically during the football World Cup. His favourite sport was horse racing. He also loved shopping and tried to buy as many magazines as he could, preferably about horses. He was proud of his possessions, but he would sometimes destroy them in a fit of anger, throwing his magazines and his television out of the bedroom window.

Childhood

Nick had spent most of his life in a large hospital for people with learning disabilities. I could only get glimpses of his childhood years, information passed on from carer to carer. Nick was an only child. His parents found him difficult, the way he would sometimes throw tantrums, scribble on the walls, throw things around the house. Mary thought he went into institutional care around the age of ten, when his parents could no longer cope with him at home. 'His parents would do everything for him,' she explained. 'They would give him anything he wanted. They never said "no" to him. So when he went into care, he was used to the world revolving around him. If you get an ice cream, you ask for another one and they won't say "no". That is why he is the way he is now. He is used to always getting what he wants.'

Nick's mother died when he was young, but his father lived into his nineties, keeping regular contact. Before he died ten years ago, he asked his partner to keep an eye on Nick for him. She agreed and became Nick's next of kin, but she didn't really want much to do with him and never visited. When Mary wrote to his stepmother to tell her that Nick had cancer, his stepmother replied that she did not want to be involved; indeed, she did not want to receive any information about him.

Nick's home and day centre

The closure of his long-stay hospital in the 1980s led to Nick's move to a newly opened residential care home, along with seven other residents. Nick didn't relate much to any of them, except to one younger man with whom he shared his bedroom and who he liked to give orders to.

Mary and her husband Alan had bought the home as a business venture from the first proprietor, and constantly struggled with the expenses of keeping up to date with new regulations and the employment of suitable staff. Apart from Helena, a support worker who had been there since the home opened and who took the residents on a toilet round before serving an early evening meal, there were a couple of young support workers with a limited command of English who had been at the home for less than six months. Mary or Alan were often present in the home, and during school holidays their three young daughters came along with them, sometimes sleeping over. The residents liked the children and missed them when they weren't there. The eight-year-old girl was particularly close to Nick, sharing his love of horses. Nick adored the girls and was always well behaved in their company. Mary would sometimes take him out with her family and never ceased to be amazed at his perfect table manners when the children were around.

Here is my first impression of Nick's home. It was 4pm, and the only members of staff were Helena and a new support worker from Eastern Europe.

Helena suggests I wait in the living room, service users (as residents seem to be called here) are just finishing their tea, they will be coming in shortly. The sitting room looks grandmotherly, with flowery carpets and rather old-fashioned decorations. It smells like it too, a musty smell that I associate with the homes of elderly people. Six armchairs and a sofa line the wall, facing a large modern television screen that is showing a children's programme.

Nick is the first to walk through the living room door. Before I can sit down next to him, several other people with learning disabilities come in. They all appear to be in their late fifties or older. I smile and shake hands with those who stop to look at me, introducing myself as Irene who has come to see Nick. Some ignore me and go straight to what is obviously 'their' chair. They all sit down, and that is basically it for the next one and a half hours

> *that I spend with them. Once, a woman is accompanied upstairs by a staff member, and brought back. Once or twice another woman leaves the room and returns. Five of the people, including Nick, do not speak at all. Nick interacts a bit with me, looking at me, responding to my signs; the others simply sit. Two men are staring at the TV. Two women sit hunched in their chairs, each apparently lost in her own world.*[2] *The other three people spend the entire time trying to tell me things* [making desperate attempts to talk to me about their lives, about family members who have died]. *They don't watch TV, but all have a colouring book and are busy with pencils. All residents seem to have severe learning disabilities, or maybe they are simply severely institutionalised...*
>
> *At the start of my visit I ask Nick about his leg, and he immediately stands up to pull his tracksuit trousers down. He strokes his left upper leg and confirms that it is painful. I urge him to put his trousers back on, as it doesn't seem appropriate for a man in his fifties to stand in his underpants in the middle of a room full of other adults. There are no staff in the room. In fact, staff rarely entered this room, except to take someone out briefly, or to intervene in a dispute.*

As the weeks went by I became more at home here, but those initial feelings of shock never left me completely. The home felt more 'homely' when Mary was around. Mary was warm and sociable, and her husband was quietly caring. For her, being here was not just a job, it was her life. She often joined the residents in the sitting room, having her cup of tea. She made an effort to get to know them and was sensitive to their needs, their life stories, their history of social deprivation. However, I often felt uncomfortable when she talked about people in the third person, as if they weren't there, discussing intimate details of their lives, including their illness and disabilities and including Nick's cancer and impending death. Mary's real love for Nick was undoubtedly crucial to him, as he had so few people in his life. But it wasn't the love of equals. As Mary struggled with grief six months after Nick's death, another resident (Ursula Smith) was dying of cancer. 'It's not easy for staff,' I pointed out to her then. 'You are not family, you are meant to be professional and cope with everything. But you were very close to Nick, and it is a loss for you.' She agreed. 'Nick and Ursula are the two people who have no family at all,' she said. 'So we are all they've got. I am very close to them. They are like my pets.'

Nick had been attending a day centre five days a week for the past 20 years. He enjoyed the routine, the activities, the staff, the buzz. In the mornings, Nick spent his days in a converted basement full of sofas, cushions, puzzles and an art room. He loved painting and would patiently and methodically cover sheet after sheet with red paint. He did not seem to have any friends. He related almost exclusively to staff, who returned his greetings and his hugs, but who then swiftly turned to other people who also needed their attention or to other staff they were chatting with.

It was a large day centre, accommodating around 150 people with learning disabilities. Although it aimed to provide meaningful day care and there were some laudable initiatives, people spent much of their time simply waiting.

> *There is an awful lot of hanging around. Lunch takes two hours; queuing and eating the food takes up to half an hour at most, so the rest of the time is left for people to do – well, nothing really… Finally, at 2pm, the afternoon activities start. Thursday is sport day. A long carpet is rolled out for boules, with chairs lined up on either side. Some people with learning disabilities take their place; others are brought or wheeled alongside. Nick soon joins them. There is another 15 minutes wait before a member of staff actually gets the balls out. One staff member then calls out each person's name in turn, starting at one end of the line of chairs, and alternating sides. Everyone gets a half-hearted clap from staff; when they hit any of the other balls, the clap is accompanied by a bit of a cheer. Hit balls are then rearranged (so it isn't clear to me whether there is actually any point in having teams). Nick soon gets up to throw a ball, but he is sent back: it isn't his turn yet. He waits another ten minutes before it gets round to his turn. He wants a ball in the colour belonging to the other team, and is told off; he only submits to throwing the right colour ball when the staff member actually sits down on the box of balls he shouldn't choose. He shows no signs of being either pleased or displeased after throwing, and goes back to his chair.*

When Nick looked thoughtful or just quiet, staff would sometimes urge him to smile. This was, if his files were to be believed, part of a 'person centred plan'. It read:

MY GOALS

1. Smile and be happy.

2. Take part in activities.
3. Learn Makaton signs: please, thank you.

Cancer

Nick was diagnosed with cancer of the bladder and was given six months to live. He eventually died 15 months after the diagnosis. During the months before the diagnosis, day centre files described an increase in disturbing behaviour – fist waving, blocking toilets with too much paper, disturbing other people's one-to-one sessions. The staff wondered whether Nick was simply bored: 'Hopefully with a fuller programme Nick's behaviour may improve.' They became worried when they noticed blood in the toilet and contacted Mary, who had made a similar discovery.

Mary described how the diagnosis was finally made. 'When we found there was blood in the toilet, we didn't know where it had come from at first. Nick has an obsession with the toilet. He always cleans himself obsessively, wiping himself, even if he hasn't done anything. He will use one toilet roll each time he goes to the toilet, and block the toilet with paper. We took him to hospital, and they did lots of tests. A scan, a cystoscopy.[3] They had to do it under general anaesthetic because he wouldn't lie still. They found a shadow. The doctor called us to say he had a massive tumour. They scraped it out via cystoscopy to stop the bleeding. But we decided not to give any radiotherapy. They would have had to give him ten or twenty doses, and he would have to go into hospital for a day and lie still for each one. He would have to lie still for ten or twenty minutes. He just couldn't do it. He had to have a bone scan, and that was very difficult, he had to lie still for that. They didn't find any spread.'

The decision not to give Nick any treatment was a difficult one, and Mary felt responsible for it. She often wondered whether she had done the right thing. Would other people have had surgery? The consultant had explained that they could remove the bladder, but this would leave Nick with a urostomy bag.[4] 'And there is absolutely no way he would have kept that on,' said Mary. 'With Nick, he likes going to the toilet, and he would still go, he wouldn't understand. I said to the consultant, "How am I going to make him understand that he needs to keep it there?" He doesn't even keep a normal catheter in.

They have tried, but he pulls them out, with balloon and all. So we felt that an operation wouldn't be good for him, he wouldn't cope very well. It is hard to make those decisions though.'

The plan now was simply to wait for symptoms to return; if they did, he would have another cystoscopy to scrape his bladder and stop the bleeding. This did indeed happen, and Nick needed to stay in hospital overnight, following the procedure under general anaesthetic. The nurse on his ward said, 'He is a real worry for us. We have talked about him so much, we've had so many meetings. He's got a nasty tumour in there. He really should have radiotherapy, but…' She made a helpless gesture, explaining that he would need daily radiotherapy treatments for a week, not to cure his cancer but to stop the bleeding. 'He would need to have a general anaesthetic, and the anaesthesist cannot stay in the radiotherapy room for a week,' the nurse explained.

Nick deteriorated gradually. He became increasingly tired and Mary would keep him at home more often. He didn't like missing the day centre though, and sometimes she wondered whether his restless and destructive behaviour (when he would soil his sheets or his clothes) was a sign of advancing illness or of protest against being kept at home. He liked to keep going with his old routines, and Mary tried as much as possible to take him out shopping or to the café, things he enjoyed, until she felt he could no longer manage it, needing to spend too much time on the toilet. In his final months, he spent most of his time at home.

Hospital

Nick already had a lot of experience with hospitals. He had often been ill, particularly with chest infections, which had landed him in intensive care on several occasions. He survived these episodes against doctors' expectations. 'He is strong, is our Nick,' Mary said.

Mary always accompanied Nick to any GP or hospital appointments, and spent most of her time with him whenever he was admitted. Her staff, she said, didn't have much of a clue, so she couldn't rely on them. Nick also demanded of her that she stayed with him in hospital: 'He won't have anyone else with him, only me, so I had to be there all the time.' Mary did not take a holiday with her family until she had ascertained that he was fairly stable and therefore unlikely to need sudden hospitalisation. She clearly needed a break but did not feel happy to take one now.

The hospital staff did not usually communicate directly with Nick. One day I accompanied Nick and Mary to hospital where he was seen in five different outpatient clinics, waiting a total of three hours, initially with much patience but then with increasing restlessness. None of the staff in the clinics spoke to him directly, except the radiographer who addressed him from behind – which he couldn't hear, because of his deafness. My notes describe the nurse who took a blood sample:

> *Like the others so far, she doesn't know how to communicate with him. She doesn't even greet him… Nick doesn't seem to notice. He simply sits where he is told, waiting for whatever is going to happen next. The nurse seems slightly nervous: 'Can he keep his arm still? He should look at you, not at his arm. Can you distract him? Make sure he doesn't use his other hand.'*

I spent a couple of hours on the ward with Nick during a hospital admission. The nurses were kind and did not seem to mind Nick wandering around, but Mary reported that it was much more difficult when there was nobody to be with him one-to-one. 'Last time he was in, he had to stay five days. The hospital expected us to stay with him, but I told them we couldn't, we don't have the staff, we have to support the other residents in the home… He is frightened in hospital, it is difficult for him. Once, I came in to visit him, and his face lit up, he clutched on to me.'

Sometimes the nurses called Mary on her mobile phone soon after she had left the ward, urging her to return just as she was picking up her children from school. Nick could be restless, pulling out his wires or tidying up other patients' medication that had arrived at the nurses' station. Mary was furious with what she saw as the hospital's lack of understanding of learning disabilities, and the nurses' demands that the support workers stayed with Nick around the clock. Usually, Nick was discharged from hospital as soon as was reasonably possible, and Mary was glad to have him back home.

Coping with cancer

The increasing levels of support Nick needed were mainly provided by Mary and Alan, probably to the detriment of the other people in the home. The demands of caring for Nick affected Mary and Alan's own family life and well-being. Mary desperately wanted to keep Nick at home; she was sure that he would not be happy or comfortable anywhere else. Having had such a difficult life, she felt that he now deserved loving care at the end of it, and only they, as his substitute family, would be able to give it. Nobody else would be as sensitive to his needs. Mary and Alan converted a downstairs room into an en-suite bedroom for him. Nick loved his new room. From now on, this was where he spent his time, content, sitting in his chair and watching the programmes he wanted to watch: horse racing, not children's television.

In his final months Nick became incontinent of urine, or maybe wet his clothes on purpose – it was hard to tell which. Mary pointed out that he used to wet his clothes if he didn't want to wear them. Now there was load after load of washing. The day centre also sent a bag full of wet clothes home each day.

The relationship between the day centre and Nick's home was somewhat strained. Mary often expressed exasperation at the day centre staff, who sent Nick home if they felt he wasn't up to attending. She didn't mind having Nick at home, but she knew Nick loved the day centre, and she saw their staff as over-anxious. As time wore on, the day centre decided that they could no longer support Nick's needs. He had already lived longer than they had anticipated. One-to-one agency staff was expensive. But mostly, they felt Nick had become too disruptive; he had broken all the cups once, and on another occasion almost threw someone off the stairs. Mary felt that such behaviour was an indication there was something not right with him. She knew that Nick missed the day centre and contemplated taking him in for visits, but decided against it. Once he was there, she would have too much difficulty convincing him to come back home with her again.

Mary often said she would do anything for Nick, anything that was needed to keep him happy and at home. But it wasn't easy. Nick needed an increasing amount of care and there was hardly any outside support. The hospice nurse visited him occasionally, but only when asked to do so. Mary and Alan rarely asked. They didn't want to bother the nurse, and sometimes months went by without contact. Mary asked social services for extra staff, but this was not forthcoming.

'I love Nick, I love him to bits,' she said. 'We don't really get enough pay for him, but I wouldn't turn him out. I should be fighting for more money. If you run a business, at the end of the day you don't want to lose money. But I don't care. I had planned to convert the downstairs bedroom with the view of having an extra resident in there. But I can't turn him out. I said to my husband, "He can't go upstairs, we just have to do it. For him…" And it is tiring. It would be nice to have a break. Then we could give some more attention to the other residents too. They have been missing out. I would like to get him into the hospice for a few days, just to give us all a break. But I want him to be at home and die here. I said to social services, "We will look after him, but I do need extra staff."'

After Nick died I spoke to someone from the social services department, as concerns had arisen about the care of Ursula Smith (see Chapter 6). 'To be honest,' she said, 'we want to work with the home, because we buy a service off them, and quite frankly, it is cheap. It would be much more expensive for us to move people out.'

Pain

Even without speech Nick had no problems explaining about the pain in his leg, gesturing at it with a screwed-up face. There were a couple of months when he had difficulty walking. Staff at home and at the day centre were sympathetic, agreeing with Nick that he was in pain, but they didn't do anything about it, apart from telling him to have a rest. They simply seemed to accept that pain was an inevitable consequence of having cancer. I intervened several times, trying to encourage Mary to liaise with the GP and the hospice nurse, who were responsible for pain assessment and the prescription of painkillers. But Mary felt she was bothering the GP enough already. She was adamant that Nick shouldn't be given morphine.[5] In her eyes, morphine was the beginning of the end. 'I will know when he cannot bear the pain any more,' she said. 'I'll give it to him when he really needs it.'

I sometimes wondered whether Nick's 'challenging behaviour' was in fact a result of unrelieved pain. Mary controlled and limited Nick's painkillers right up to his final weeks. 'We give him co-codamol,' she said, 'but not all the time, not every four hours as it says on the box, but only if he needs it.'

Nick was in hospital for a couple of days, a few weeks before he died. Mary explained how wonderful the effect of morphine had been: 'They just said, "Right, we are going to give him something for the pain" and they gave him morphine. I am telling you, within ten minutes he was a different man. He was sitting up, talking, much more cheerful. It was amazing.' Despite this positive experience, she remained reluctant to give him morphine at home.

Nick's understanding

Nick didn't understand that he had cancer or was terminally ill, and staff at the day centre and at his home agreed that this lack of understanding was a good thing. The support workers were convinced that it protected him from worrying about the illness, and may even have protected him from an early death. He just kept going as if there was nothing wrong. Mary was clear that she wouldn't tell him; she herself wouldn't want to know that she was dying either.

Nick seemed to cope with the increasing tiredness by simply taking himself off for a rest when he needed to, or putting his head on his arms for a snooze, ready for action again when he woke. He never questioned his support workers about why he needed to be in hospital, although he wanted their support. There was, in Nick's case, no 'conspiracy of silence', probably because his deafness and the general lack of meaningful communication with him confined him to a silent world anyway.

Nick's house mates were not explicitly told, but Mary talked freely about Nick's cancer with me in their presence, as if they weren't there. Some had good verbal understanding, and I sometimes wondered what they thought of it all. They never asked any questions. Mary didn't think they would miss Nick after he died. 'He isn't very nice to them.'

Dying and beyond

Nick's final hospitalisation came after he suddenly collapsed at home. Mary thought he was dying there and then, and rang an ambulance. Doctors suspected a heart attack. 'He stayed five days,' Mary said. 'In the end they said, "There is nothing really we are doing for him here, could you take him home please?" So I did.'

Nick had a gentle time at home, often sitting in the kitchen where Mary was drinking tea or Alan was doing the administration. He bought bunches of flowers for his room and proudly showed them to me. He gradually spent more time in bed, until it became clear that he was going to die. Mary later described his last day:

> 'The day before was terrible. He was so restless. He just couldn't sit still, he was up and down, sitting on the floor, taking his clothes off, lashing out to people... It wasn't like him. I was really panicking, I kept ringing and ringing the hospice nurse for advice. She came immediately and said, 'I know you don't want to hear this, but I think it is best to put up a syringe driver[6] and sedate him.' After that he just went to sleep. We put him in his bed. I stayed with him for a bit, but I couldn't look at him. He was just like a body, an empty shell, not him, just a body breathing. So I went home. My daughter was with him, she was sleeping on Nick's stomach. I said, 'What are you doing?' and she said, 'I'm just resting my head on him, look, it is OK, he is still breathing.' She is eight years old. In the night Nick's breathing changed, and they called me, so I came. I sat with him when he died. He took his last breath at 5.40am. Then I closed his eyes and tried to close his mouth. We washed him, put him in pyjamas. They didn't want us to get him dressed yet, so I put pyjamas on him. We gave him his last wash. He looked really peaceful. It was nice, you know? Then they came and took him away... I don't think he wanted to die. I think he was fighting it. He loved his life. Even if he couldn't do much, he loved it, just being around, sitting there, going out, his day centre, his cups of tea...'

As Nick had no family to organise his funeral, it was organised by Mary and paid for by the local council. A sign at the crematorium announced the funeral of 'Nicolas Ballard' (rather than 'Nicholas') at 10am. All Nick's house mates came, as well as some people from his day centre. Nick's stepmother and some of her relatives were there, too. Although I didn't ask her, she tried to explain to me why she hadn't visited Nick. 'I did send Christmas cards, but he was well cared for...' The tributes described Nick as a happy man who loved life.

Mary was taken aback by the strength of her grief. 'He is constantly on my mind,' she sobbed. 'I think of him when I close my eyes and I still think of him when I open them. I dream about him. Other people who have died are there too, my father and mother. I need to clear out his room but I can't do it. I had to go in there to throw away his flowers because they had died...and taking out his clothes...it is as if I am killing him again.'

During the months that followed Mary tried to remain professional. She was preoccupied by financial worries – Nick's death had left her with a gap in her income – and busied herself with the running of her home, not allowing herself to dwell on Nick too much. But she often found herself talking about him, and acknowledged that her closeness to him meant that she was grieving. It was almost unbearably difficult when she had to live through similar emotions when, six months later, she supported Ursula Smith who also died of cancer. She did not have any support in this bereavement, except from her husband.

'I think of Nick, you know?' she said, nine months after his death. 'All the time, I am thinking...did we do the right thing? Did we do everything that was possible?'

CHAPTER 2

Diagnosis and Treatment

Cancer affects all of us. One in three people in the UK will get cancer in their lifetime. More than one in four people will die of cancer. Unfortunately, there are no firm figures available to tell us exactly what the cancer risk is for people with learning disabilities, but there are clear indications that the number of people with learning disabilities who develop cancer is rising (Hogg and Tuffrey-Wijne 2008). Most of the studies so far have looked at people living in institutions, and found a relatively low cancer incidence (Cooke 1997). More recent studies of people with learning disabilities living in the community found that their risk of cancer is similar to that of the rest of the population, although some of these studies come from outside the UK (Janicki *et al.* 2002; Patja, Mölsä and Iivanainen 2001). A study of death certificates in London found that cancer was recorded as the cause of death for 16 per cent of people with learning disabilities (Hollins *et al.* 1998). It may well be that the true risk of cancer for people with learning disabilities is higher than those studies suggest: some cancer deaths may not be recorded or reported as such, and some cancers may not be diagnosed.

One thing is clear. Learning disability services will find that more and more of their clients develop cancer, and cancer services will see growing numbers of people with learning disabilities coming through their doors. The risk of most types of cancer increases with age, and people with learning disabilities are living longer than ever before.

What is also clear is that many people with learning disabilities will be affected by cancer at some point in their lives, either because they develop the disease themselves, or because someone close to them does. Nine people in the Veronica Project had lost one or both parents to cancer, and most had other relatives who had suffered the same fate.

This chapter looks at how people's cancer diagnosis was made, how the cancer progressed, what cancer treatments were offered, how such treatment decisions were taken, and how the men and women coped with all this. I will start by introducing Lily Lamb.

Lily Lamb

Lily Lamb was 55 years old. The limitations posed on her by her moderate learning disabilities were exacerbated by her speech impediment. Although she could speak in full sentences, even those who knew her well often struggled to understand what she was saying; as a consequence she often stuck to single words or short, simple sentences. She preferred to sit quietly and watch what was going on rather than joining in with people's conversation, to the point of seeming rude.

Fifteen years ago Lily moved from the home of her parents into a residential care home, where she now lived with six other people with learning disabilities. When I asked her what she liked doing most, she said without hesitation, 'Meetings. Taking decisions.' Lily had a lifelong desire to be in control of her situation, and a lifelong fear of being abandoned. She loved pretty things, nice clothes, the colour purple. She wanted to look nice but was self-conscious about her weight, her excess facial hair and her poor speech. She lacked confidence and self-esteem. She often asked her carers, 'Am I a good girl?'

Cancer

Lily was diagnosed with cancer 18 months after her father's death. It is not clear who first noticed that anything was wrong. With hindsight, Lily's support workers realised that the signs of tiredness they had attributed to a delayed grief reaction were probably an early symptom of cancer. Lily started complaining of painful legs, but she had arthritis, and her legs had been intermittently painful for years. Nobody thought much of it, although there were a few visits to the GP. Two years after her death, Lily's family were still upset that the support workers had told her to exercise, to get up, to walk everywhere, over-riding Lily's protests that 'I can't'. Her brother Bob and his wife May deeply resented the fact that Lily had been in terrible pain and had complained of her pain, yet was not sent to hospital for several months.

Bob sounded the alarm bells on his return from holiday. He hadn't seen Lily for a while, and now he could see a change in her. He felt that something was seriously wrong. Whenever Lily visited him and his wife May, she complained of pain. One week it was her legs; another week it was her upper arms. May thought it wasn't right to keep giving Lily paracetamol and insisted that Bob spoke to the support workers. Lily had rarely complained of pain in the past, not unless the pain was really quite bad; and now the complaints were constant. In the end it was Fiona, the day centre manager, who took action. By now, Lily could barely walk. Fiona recalled how it had taken her two hours to walk home from the day centre, despite it being only a street away. When Lily couldn't get out of her chair, Fiona called an ambulance. Tests revealed stomach cancer with extensive spread into her bones. No cancer treatments were given; it was too late for that. The aim now was to keep Lily comfortable.

In the following month, whilst Lily was in hospital, a hairline fracture was found in her hip, but the hospital did not relay this information to the family and support workers. The hospital staff encouraged Lily to exercise with her zimmer frame to prepare her for managing the stairs, and she was sent back home to climb the flight of stairs to her bedroom. It took an hour of excruciating pain to get there. She never walked properly again.

Despite their feelings of distress at the missed opportunities for an earlier diagnosis, Bob and May pondered: 'If we had found it three months earlier, what difference would that have made? It would still have been too late.'

Lily struggled with pain throughout her illness, even during the weeks leading up to her death, nine weeks after I first met her. She was, by then, in a hospice where the staff promptly gave her extra morphine whenever she complained of pain. Her family was convinced that the memory of the unrecognised, almost unbearable pain she had been in at the beginning of her illness prevented her from being completely pain free now. I wondered whether her pain stemmed not only from the cancer itself, but also from a painful life, as had been the case with Vincent Sweeney. Her inner turmoil was obvious from my very first meeting with her, when she had just arrived home from hospital. 'I've got pain,' she repeated again and again, grabbing hold of my hand and locking her eyes into mine. 'I should be in hospital. I've got pain.' She was silent for a while, then looked into my eyes again: 'It is not my fault.'

Later, she continued to seek reassurance from the hospice nurses, the way she had from her carers in the past. 'I'm not naughty,' she said when she needed them, as if trying to convince herself as well as the nurses. 'Are you cross with me? I'm a good girl, aren't I?'

The cancer diagnosis

Cancers of the breast and lung are among the most common types of cancer, and this was reflected in the Veronica Project. Three men had lung cancer; three women had breast cancer. Others had cancers that had started in the bowel, stomach, bladder, penis, and testicles. One person had lymphoma; for another it was never discovered where the cancer started, only that it had spread. Spread of cancer to other parts of the body was found in eight of the people.

The cancer diagnosis was made before I met any of the study participants. To establish how the diagnosis was made in each case, I had to rely on what was written in the files and on what people remembered.

The events that generally prompt people to seek medical help are different for each kind of cancer. They may be subjective feelings or symptoms, such as pain or tiredness; or observable signs: a lump, blood in the stool, coughing, shortness of breath. Before a diagnosis can be made, such symptoms must be reported, or the signs observed by the patient or carer.

For the ten cases where I could establish the course of events, the problems were recognised late in the illness for a variety of reasons. I found problems with both the noticing and the reporting, but I also found that in some cases the reported symptoms were not believed. It is difficult to say whether this resulted in a death that might have been prevented – although in some cases, such as John Davies', this was probably so. The fact remains that Lily was not the only person whose cancer was already so far advanced that, by the time the diagnosis was made, it was too late for curative treatment.

The patient did not complain

John Davies was the most striking example of a patient whose lack of complaints had far-reaching consequences. He used elaborate strategies to hide his symptoms. In other cases, symptoms had to get to the point where a carer noticed and was concerned enough to take action.

One of the women, Ursula Smith, who had severe learning disabilities, was diagnosed with breast cancer 14 years ago. She had responded well to treatment at the time, and people thought she was cured. Mary, her home manager, became concerned when Ursula began to have falls, one of which resulted in a broken arm: 'She basically stopped walking. That wasn't normal. So I took her to the doctor and said, "Look, she is not moving around, can you do some tests?"' It transpired that Ursula's cancer had spread to her bones. She died two months later; she only complained of pain during those final few months.

Noticing the signs of illness is especially important when people lack the ability to complain in words. People with severe and profound learning disabilities are often totally dependent on their carers to act as a bridge with the health care professionals. Dimas Ferreira, for example, had very severe learning disabilities and communicated by making noises. It will never be known how long he had cancer before one of his carers noticed an unusual lump at the side of Dimas' neck. The lump turned out to be a cancer that had spread to his lymphatic system; the source of the cancer was never found.

The carers misinterpreted behavioural changes

Nick Ballard, who had severe learning disabilities and didn't speak, was taken to the doctor when carers noticed blood in the toilet, but this followed months of increasingly disturbed behaviour. It can be very difficult, even for the most dedicated and observant carers, to attribute such behaviour correctly to an underlying physical problem. Most staff working in learning disability services are poorly trained and do not have a background in health care. An estimated 75 per cent of the learning disability workforce is unqualified (Department of Health 2001a).

Physical discomfort can be expressed in widely varying ways, including behavioural changes that could be seen as 'challenging'. In an earlier study (Tuffrey-Wijne 2002) a man with a liver condition from which he later died became incontinent of faeces, but the staff in his residential home thought that he was 'playing up', soiling himself to annoy them. When his condition deteriorated, staff saw it as manipulation. It wasn't until his skin turned yellow that they took him to the doctor. It is only with hindsight that such carers understood the significance of some behaviours, often with guilt and self-reproach: 'We should have picked that up earlier.'

There were several instances of 'diagnostic overshadowing', where someone's behaviour was attributed to the learning disability itself, rather than to a physical cause.

Marion Prentice had Down's syndrome, severe learning disabilities and limited speech. Her diagnosis of breast cancer came after her support worker noticed, when helping her wash, that her nipple was inverted. A week later the nipple was bleeding. When the support worker checked Marion's breast and felt a lump she took her to the GP immediately. She reflected:

> 'Looking back, we can see now that there were so many different ways in which Marion was trying to tell us that she wasn't well, before her diagnosis. That there was something wrong with her breast. We just didn't pick it up. When she was on holiday, she sat down in the middle of the road. She wouldn't normally do that. She does sometimes have challenging behaviour, but not like that. And the other thing was, she kept touching the breasts of another woman in the house. And we just said to her that she shouldn't do it. We just told Marion off for touching her in that way, but now you look back and you think, my goodness, she was trying to tell us that there was something wrong with her breasts!'

The patient was not believed

Vincent Sweeney complained so much about so many aspects of his life that his family had stopped taking him seriously. Complaints were just seen as part of his personality. Lily Lamb's complaints of pain were also not taken seriously at first. This was perhaps more surprising, as Lily did not usually complain of pain; in fact, she had always been highly reluctant to take paracetamol or aspirin, and her readiness to take them now rang alarm bells with her family.

It may well be that some people indicate physical discomfort in order to get attention, but even when such complaints do not have a strictly physical cause, the need for attention is real. The complaints may be the only way someone knows of communicating his or her needs. Vincent himself was aware of this: 'I tell them that I am having pain. I'm not in pain really, I am just lonely and worried.' It is important that any complaints of physical discomfort are taken seriously, and all possible causes investigated.

Doctors did not make the diagnosis immediately

In some cases, the cancer diagnosis was made swiftly. Marion Prentice's signs of breast cancer were unambiguous enough. However, in several other cases the GP didn't immediately refer the patient for further tests. John Davies was initially sent home with the message that he had a urine infection. He never went back to his doctor. Such initial mis-diagnosis can happen to anybody, not only to people with learning disabilities; but it may be much harder for people with learning disabilities, particularly those who do not have carers to support them and advocate for them, to decide that the doctor may have been wrong.

Amanda Cresswell's persistence with her GP was impressive. She explained:

> 'I was starting to feel unwell. I had no energy, I felt really tired, I kept drinking more than usual, and I just wanted to go and have a good sleep... So I went to the doctor, and he said, "Oh, there's nothing wrong with you." He couldn't find anything that was wrong with me, and I *knew* there was something wrong, because every time I went up the stairs I was having problems breathing. I had this cough, and this cough was a bit

like whooping cough. I went back to the doctor, and he kept saying there's nothing wrong, but I knew… I still wasn't feeling right, I wasn't eating properly, I lost a lot of weight. I went back to my doctor with my social worker, and he *still* said, "There's nothing wrong with you."'

Amanda was eventually diagnosed with lymphoma after she collapsed and was taken to hospital. She was successfully treated, but five years later she was still angry about the disbelieving doctor.

People who live in residential care services usually depend on staff to advocate for them. Sometimes the carers, too, need to be persistent before getting a diagnosis. Dimas Ferreira's carers were told by a hospital consultant that the neck lump was just fatty tissue: no cause for concern. They weren't convinced; they kept a close eye on the lump and found that it grew overnight. They took him back to his GP the following day, and further tests confirmed cancer.

Pete Carpenter's support workers took him to the doctor a number of times during the months leading up to his diagnosis of lung cancer. Pete had severe learning disabilities and could not indicate clearly what was wrong with him, but his carers were concerned about his weight loss and coughing.

Worries about symptoms after the cancer diagnosis

Once the cancer diagnosis was made, most carers were on the alert for further signs and symptoms. This brought new anxieties. Changes in behaviour were particularly worrying. Was this anything to do with the cancer, or was it something more innocent? When was the cancer time bomb going to explode?

Ben Edwards had advanced prostate cancer, and Yanna, his home manager, struggled with understanding his behaviour throughout his illness:

'He is challenging. He got very angry a couple of times. Twice he hit a resident, and once he lashed out at staff… I'm not sure what it is. He has been like this before, it isn't completely new behaviour, but it has never been this bad. I am giving him the benefit of doubt. I think it has something to do with his cancer. It must be. I don't know, I just think it must be making him feel different, and he can't express it.'

Carers didn't have a clear understanding of the likely course of the illness, and this made them anxious about what was happening. A concerned support worker at Nick Ballard's day centre said:

> 'We were told that he had six months to live, but that has now gone, and he seems to be doing well. I don't know what to expect. He just had a blackout, and I don't know about blackouts. Could the cancer have spread to his brain?'

Before the cancer diagnosis, there was a tendency to attribute signs and symptoms to other causes; but after the cancer diagnosis, carers suspected that any changes were due to the cancer. They had little support from health care staff to guide them through their worries; even those with supportive GPs hesitated to contact them. Ben's home manager said: 'I don't want to go to the GP too often, you know? I don't want to keep bothering them. They have been very good about it, but still.'

Cancer treatments

Many cancer treatments are not easy to cope with. Surgery, radiotherapy and chemotherapy all come at a considerable physical and emotional cost to the patient. There are repeated trips to hospital, waits in waiting rooms, seemingly endless tests, needles, intimidating equipment, needing to take your clothes off, to put unfamiliar garments on, to lie still, to take unpleasant medications... And all of this has no immediate positive outcome. Patients who have undergone treatments may feel more ill, nauseous or tired. Their hair may fall out. Surgery may leave them with a urinary catheter or a colostomy bag, with painful wounds, with the loss of a body part.

Tests for cancer can be equally challenging. An accurate cancer diagnosis usually depends on the results of medical investigations: scans, biopsies, explorations with cameras into the lungs, bowels or bladder. Diagnostic tests are more difficult to cope with if people don't understand what they are for, if they find it hard to lie still, or if they are frightened.

Cancer treatments can either be given in the hope that they will bring a cure or at least prolong someone's life (curative treatment), or to relieve symptoms (palliative treatment). Decisions about cancer treatments can be difficult, because it is not always clear beforehand whether or not the treatment will be successful. Treatments may work in some patients but not in others. They may relieve symptoms, or they may not. The question whether the benefits of treatment outweigh the drawbacks is a personal one, but in order to make that decision, patients and their families need to have information from someone who can explain the options clearly, usually their doctor or specialist nurse. Such information needs to consist not only of what might happen if the treatment is given, but also of what is likely to happen if the treatment is *not* given. Carers of people with learning disabilities may worry, with good reason, that the person will not cope with treatment; but the effects of non-treatment must also be considered and clearly spelled out. Dying of untreated cancer is not necessarily the easiest option.

This was illustrated poignantly by Linda McEnhill, who described the case of a woman with learning disabilities in her sixties who had breast cancer. The woman was frightened of operations and had refused surgery. She was quite clear about this refusal and it was documented in her notes. She was treated with medication instead. However, when the cancer progressed she asked, 'This lump in my breast is growing, it won't kill me, will it?' It seems that she had not understood the implications of her refusal (McEnhill 2008, p.160).

Some symptoms of cancer, including some types of pain, can be treated effectively. Mary, the home manager for Ursula Smith whose breast cancer had spread to her bones, was impressed by the impact of a single dose of radiotherapy: 'It has done wonders. She was in *so* much pain. She was in agony. You couldn't touch her. And no way would she walk. But now, she is fine, she even gets up and walks sometimes.' For Ursula, radiotherapy had been worth it.

Decisions about tests and treatment are usually complex. They can be even more difficult for people with learning disabilities, who may need more help to understand and to cope. Whether or not tests and treatments were given, and how people coped, depended on a range of factors. The ability to understand was one important factor, but it wasn't the only one.

Being given information and choice

Without clear information and understanding, it would probably be more difficult for most of us to cope with cancer treatments. However, very few people in the Veronica Project were given clear information. When they were, it did indeed help them to cope.

Amanda Cresswell had mild learning disabilities. Her mother had died of a brain tumour when she was in her teens. Amanda was diagnosed with lymphoma, and she coped with months of radiotherapy and chemotherapy because her doctor had given her a clear choice. She remembered:

> 'There were lots of meetings. It was good that they explained all my options to me. I had to have a big meeting with the family I was living with at the time, and my social workers, and my doctor said, "If you don't have chemotherapy, within three days you could be dead." And he asked me what I wanted. I said to him, "I don't want to die like my mum, it was too late to save my mum, and I'm too young to die." I was only 30 years old. I knew I didn't want to die. I knew that I wanted to live. I was thinking of my mum then.'

Pauline Deweert, who had moderate learning disabilities, described her cancer and treatment in very practical terms. When surgeons had removed the cancer from her breast, she insisted on seeing it. Five years later, she still shuddered at the thought and described it to me repeatedly:

> 'I wanted to look at it. It was black. I didn't like it. Shall I tell you what it was like? It was long like a sausage. All black. It was oozing, and smelly. I didn't like that. I didn't like smelling. I could smell it. It made me feel funny. It made me go all cold inside.'

The memory of that 'black sausage' helped Pauline to attend her follow-up appointments and to take her medication (Tamoxifen). 'I don't want it to come back,' she said. Pauline was given a choice of treatments. She explained, waving big circles in the air at the memory: 'I could have radiotherapy or chemotherapy. Chemotherapy makes your hair fall out, and I didn't like the sound of that. So I chose radiotherapy. You go in a machine, it goes round and round.'

Amanda Cresswell was keen to give her advice to doctors and nurses.

> 'It is important to explain exactly what is going to happen. Like if you are giving radiotherapy, wherever you need to have it, they mark it with a cross, and then you lay on a bed, and then they do the radiation, and that would make sure all the cancer cells had gone. And if they give you chemotherapy, tell them how long they're going to have it for and what's going to happen. When I started having chemotherapy, they said that my body's going to change, and I might be a bit moody sometimes. And they were right. I was getting really bad hot flushes sometimes, one minute I was hot, one minute I was cold... But at least they told you about that beforehand, and that definitely helped. Because if I hadn't known, then I would have thought, "Oh my goodness, what's going on here?"'

Marion Prentice's carers were highly creative in helping Marion to understand and cope with surgery for breast cancer. It was a challenge to support Marion: she didn't like change, she didn't like the unfamiliar, and her learning disabilities were severe – she couldn't understand abstract concepts. Marion's learning disability nurse asked the hospital exactly what was going to happen, and produced a resource consisting of photographs that showed the sequence of events for the mastectomy. Marion's support worker explained:

> 'It even had a photo of the stockings she would have to put on. So we could go through it: "Look, here is the hospital, you are going to go into the hospital, take your clothes off, get into bed, you will have an injection, put the stockings on," etc. So I could sit next to her and point: "Look, you've had your stockings on, next you are going to go into a different room for the operation." I told her again and again about her breast. How it was bad. She could see that, because it was bleeding, and she absolutely hates mess. And how they were going to take the bad breast off. She was fine with that too. She didn't want a messy breast.'

A similar personalised resource was produced to help Marion cope with the follow-up mammograms. It was time-consuming, but it paid off. Marion was successfully treated, and by the time I started visiting her, almost a year after the diagnosis, cancer no longer affected her daily life. Later, she began to show symptoms of dementia and was diagnosed with Alzheimer's disease. The illness advanced quickly, and three years after the cancer diagnosis she died in a nursing home far away from her family and friends, not of cancer but of heart failure.

Carers need to understand what is happening

Carers will only be able to support people in the way Marion's support workers did if they themselves know and understand what is happening. Some support workers, including home managers, found themselves struggling to get the information they needed. On a number of occasions, their understanding of the cancer was rather vague. Ben Edwards had testicular cancer, but some of his support workers gave me confusing information, leaving me unsure whether his cancer was actually in his testicle, or in his stomach, or in his prostate. They weren't sure either.

When Pete Carpenter was in hospital for a bronchoscopy[7] under local anaesthetic, the two support workers who had come with him from his residential care home didn't know what to expect. They were asked to step out of the way by a nurse who rushed in to stick wires onto Pete's chest for an electro-cardiogram (ECG). They were shocked to find that they were not allowed to stay with Pete during the procedure, as had been the case during previous investigations. They lacked the confidence to remonstrate with the hospital staff, and felt helpless as they sat in the hospital coffee shop while Pete was in theatre. They knew that Pete was worried and uncomfortable, but would the nurses know it, too? The nurses had seemed unaware of the anxiety that his carers could see underneath his co-operative exterior. When Pete returned to the ward, he looked pale and anxious; his face split open into a huge smile when he saw his support workers. Waiting for discharge, the support workers had no idea what was going to happen next. Some questions they asked ('Can Pete have a bath tonight?') received conflicting answers. Clearly, in such circumstances, it is difficult for carers to prepare people for a hospital procedure or to provide them with sensitive support.

Several home managers felt that it was a huge effort to get information from the hospital. Mary, who supported first Nick Ballard and then Ursula Smith, said:

> 'It would really help to know exactly what was happening. It was so difficult to get any information out of the doctors in the hospital. I just wanted to know what was going on, so that I could make decisions. I would have taken her home if I'd known [that she was dying]. And the nurses wouldn't tell me anything. They would say, "Ask the doctor," but then the doctor wouldn't be around for three or four hours, and when he did come he would say, "It might be a chest infection." How difficult is that to figure out? Why couldn't the nurses have told me that?'

In order to provide adequate information and support to someone with learning disabilities, co-operation, thoughtfulness and compassion are needed from the hospital staff who do know what is going to happen, as well as from the social care staff who have an intimate knowledge of the person's needs.

Turning treatment into a routine

Most people with learning disabilities are no strangers to hospital. Cancer is often not the first medical condition they've suffered from. Some people with learning disabilities are frightened of hospitals or have a needle phobia, but this was not the case for anyone in the Veronica Project. Some people positively enjoyed the contact with doctors and nurses. For others, hospital was a welcome outing. If hospital appointments, treatments or tests had to be endured regularly, they could be turned into a new routine, and this could in itself be an effective way of helping someone cope.

Ben Edwards had just a few passions in life. He loved buying videos, and he loved his food. As luck would have it, the hospital where he had to go for regular check-ups and scans had a charity shop that sold videos. He enjoyed his hospital appointments. His carers told him that they were off to the hospital shop to buy a video, followed by lunch at the hospital café, and Ben saw this as the real purpose of the trip; the appointment with the doctor was just an annoying hold-up. He got to know the nurses and underwent the scans without any difficulties, keen to get it over and done with.

Not coping with tests and treatments

With good information or careful preparation, several people coped well with tests and treatments; but sometimes medical procedures were tried and abandoned, because the patient had been too uncooperative or too frightened.

Vincent Sweeney needed a scan to discover whether the cancer had spread, but he found it too frightening. He said:

> 'My family want me to have it. But I just couldn't. You have to go in a tunnel, a machine like that, and they put a needle in your arm, like that, with dye in it. I just couldn't do it. I went back another time to try again, but when they put me on the bed I just said no. My family were angry, they were shouting at me that I was wasting their time.'

Vincent finally managed to have the scan when the whole procedure was carefully explained to him, and he was given medication to help him relax.

Treatment decisions were often taken by carers

Very few people in the Veronica Project were given full and clear information. In most cases, they were not involved in treatment decisions. This study was undertaken before the Mental Capacity Act passed into English law (Department for Constitutional Affairs 2007), which includes an obligation for doctors to give information about treatment in a format the patient can understand. I will describe this in more detail in the next chapter. Most of the people with learning disabilities were not included in decision making, usually because they were deemed to lack the capacity to understand or to cope. Sometimes, doctors and families or social care staff discussed this together, but there were also instances where doctors simply complied with carers' wishes. They did not question a carer's assessment that someone 'just couldn't cope with the treatments', they didn't explore further options for involvement, nor did they carry out an assessment of capacity to understand.

The decision not to give Nick Ballard an operation that would leave him with a permanent catheter was based on Mary's assessment that he would not be able to keep the catheter in. This may well have been an accurate assessment. However, he would have benefited from radiotherapy, which was not given because the staff thought he wouldn't be able to lie still. Radiotherapy would have been an important treatment in his case. Nick liked routines, he was used to hospital, and he was used to being told what to do. It was therefore not inconceivable that, with dedicated preparation and commitment from his daily carers and from the hospital staff, he might have coped with a course of radiotherapy.

There were a few cases where a 'best interest meeting' was held to decide about treatment. When the question arose whether Ben Edwards should have chemotherapy, the hospital organised a meeting with the medical team, Ben's home manager Yanna and several members of Ben's family. The outcome was that the possible benefits of treatment did not justify the burden for Ben, and therefore he would not be given chemotherapy. His brother explained:

> 'I was glad Yanna was there. We really listened to her. She was very good. She didn't say, "This is what I think," she said, "This is what I feel." She felt it was too much for Ben to be put through all the chemo. I think about 90 per cent of our decision was based on her. We trusted her. And then the doctor explained about numbers, chances and so on, and that was very helpful. That steered us towards the decision. I am happy with the decision we took.'

In several cases there was no such 'best interest meeting' involving medical staff, social care staff and relatives. Instead, doctors relied on the carers to direct them; but carers' views were sometimes based on their own opinions, rather than on an assessment of what might be best for the person or of what the person might want. One of Marion Prentice's support workers said: 'If the doctors said that there was a 50/50 chance of the treatments working, then I would say: forget it. Just let her be happy.'

Marion was lucky to have other support workers who committed themselves to helping her cope with her mastectomy, but the comment is significant nevertheless. Most patients will probably choose to put up with the unpleasantness of treatments if they know that they can save or prolong their life. Given a 50 per cent chance of success (or even a 10 per cent chance of success) most of us would probably opt to have the treatment. Why, then, would this be different for people with learning disabilities?

'Quality of life' was, quite rightly, an important consideration in treatment decisions. However, it was not always clear whether a non-treatment decision was based on a careful consideration of patients' quality of life *from their own perspective.*

When Dimas Ferreira's cancer was diagnosed, it was incurable, but the doctors proposed a course of radiotherapy treatment in order to prolong his life. Dimas was 47 and had profound learning disabilities. His next of kin was his elderly aunt, Mrs Lopez, who had been visiting him for the past 14 years – before that, his grandmother used to visit. Mrs Lopez did not think Dimas should be put through the pain and distress of treatment. He greatly disliked hospitals, and she didn't feel he would be able to understand. What was the point of prolonging his life and making him suffer? The doctors went along with her decision and sent Dimas back to his residential home. He died nine months later.

There is no doubt that Dimas lacked capacity to take decisions about his treatment and care. The Mental Capacity Act (Department for Constitutional Affairs 2007) stresses that when decisions have to be made about life-sustaining treatment, people must not make assumptions about the person's quality of life. A government document on working with people with learning disabilities who lack capacity to consent to treatment states that 'you should use the person's ordinary life with their disability as the baseline from which to judge whether treatment will impose excessive burdens on them' (Department of Health 2001b, p.18). Such situations are always difficult, as Mary said about the non-treatment decisions taken for Nick: 'We felt that an operation wouldn't be good for him, he wouldn't cope very well. It is hard to make those decisions though.'

Most carers, whether they are relatives or paid carers, are compassionate and want to do the best for the person. However, it is possible that they don't fully appreciate the value people with learning disabilities may place on their own lives, and they fail to see their capacity to cope. Carers should always ask themselves whether they have tried everything possible to support the person and to enable him or her to cope with treatment.

Carers' suspicions of unfair treatment

It wasn't always the case that carers preferred non-treatment. In several instances, carers were highly suspicious of the fact that someone wasn't offered treatment. They wondered whether the person was being discriminated against because of his or her learning disabilities, and needed to be reassured that this was not the case.

Richard Horwood had mild learning disabilities and lived independently with a friend, supported by a team of staff. He attended a day centre several times a week. When he was diagnosed with lung cancer, staff at the day centre expressed their concern. One support worker said: 'I'm not sure they are giving him the most aggressive treatments available. If it was me, I would want all the treatment I could get.' Richard's learning disability nurse was able to discuss this with the hospital consultant and was reassured that treatments were not given, not because of his learning disabilities, but because they were unlikely to be effective. His cancer was too far advanced.

Doctors may have taken non-treatment decisions based on their knowledge that treatment would be futile, and not on an under-rating of the quality of life of someone with disabilities; but they did not always communicate this clearly with the carers.

Mary, the manager of Nick and Ursula's home, felt she had to advocate strongly for her clients' rights: 'I'm worried that people give up on her. They hear she's got cancer, and they give up... She has nobody to fight for her, so *I've* got to fight. The GP shouldn't give up on her.'

There did, however, seem to be some instances where people were not offered the same kinds of interventions as the general population. The three women with breast cancer had all undergone surgery, and because they all had large breasts, this was obvious to anyone looking carefully, even when they were dressed. Marion Prentice's support workers decided not to attend an appointment to fit a prosthesis, as Marion found it very difficult to attend hospital appointments, and she already had to cope with numerous other appointments that affected her health directly. 'Of all the things she needed to see doctors for, or go to hospital, that seemed the least urgent,' her support worker said. She then pondered:

> 'But what I find strange is that they haven't offered her a breast reconstruction. I mean, surely if you or I had a breast removed, we would have been offered that, standard. Why not her? They just think, "Oh, she is not a sexual person, it is not important." It's not right that she wasn't offered a reconstruction.'

These women may well have benefited from a breast reconstruction. Pauline Deweert worried greatly about her appearance. She liked looking nice and smelling nice.

> 'I don't wear a bra. Do you think I should? Is it all right? They were going to put something inside the breast to make it bigger, but they didn't do it. So now it is smaller. Is it all right? Do you notice it?'

Summary

Late diagnosis

The cancer diagnosis was delayed for most people with learning disabilities, for a variety of reasons:

- People did not complain of any symptoms. One man, who had good verbal skills, tried to hide his symptoms. Others with more severe learning disabilities did not complain of subjective symptoms such as pain; therefore, the diagnosis could not be made until there were observable signs, such as a lump.
- The carers misinterpreted behavioural changes. Some people's behaviour before the cancer diagnosis could, on reflection, be interpreted as a way of communicating physical discomfort; however, at the time, carers had thought that it was challenging behaviour related to the learning disability itself ('diagnostic overshadowing').
- People were not believed: their complaints of pain were dismissed by family or carers.

- Doctors did not make the diagnosis immediately. Some people and/or their carers needed to be persistent, going back to the doctor several times before an accurate diagnosis was made. At least one person believed that his doctor's initial mis-diagnosis was correct, and did not go back when his symptoms worsened.
- Once the cancer diagnosis was made, many carers worried and were unsure whether or not to attribute new signs and symptoms to cancer.

Cancer treatments

Whether or not tests and treatments were given depended on a range of factors.

- Very few people were given full information and choice about treatments. Those who were given clear information appreciated this; it helped them to make a choice and subsequently to cope with the treatments. They wanted simple, clear and unambiguous information. One woman with severe learning disabilities was helped by careful preparation and information at each step of the treatment.
- Carers did not always understand the diagnosis, the investigations or the treatment. This made it difficult for them to give adequate support to the person with learning disabilities. Sometimes hospital staff failed to explain to the person and carers what was happening or what to expect.
- Some people got used to visiting hospital for tests or treatments. These could be turned into a routine that made them easier to cope with. It helped to have familiar hospital staff.
- Several people coped well with tests and treatments, but some didn't. Uncooperative behaviour or fear meant that some tests and treatments could not be given.
- Most treatment decisions were heavily influenced by the opinions of the family or residential care staff. In most cases, doctors relied on the carers and did not make an independent assessment of the patient's capacity to contribute to the

decision making process. An assessment of 'quality of life' was important in such decisions, but in some cases, such assessment may not have taken full account of the patient's own perspective.

- In some cases, carers were suspicious of doctors' non-treatment decisions, wondering whether the person was discriminated against because of his or her learning disabilities.

CHAPTER 3

Truth-telling and Understanding

'What is going on? What is happening to me?' These were questions in the minds of several men and women. Vincent Sweeney, for example, worried about this constantly. It was also an issue for almost all the carers. 'Should we tell him? What should we tell? How should we tell? Who should tell?'

This chapter explores what 'truth-telling' means. I will describe in detail what happened: how much people were (or weren't) helped to understand about their cancer, how much they *did* understand, and how they coped with this. I will focus on the story of Sally Burnett in some detail, as issues about truth-telling and understanding were paramount in her situation. But first of all, here is what happened with Lily Lamb.

Lily Lamb's understanding of cancer

Lily had not been told that she had cancer when she was first diagnosed, but when she came home from hospital, her brother Bob decided that the time had come for him to tell her the truth. She had been wondering what was happening to her. 'Something is not right,' she said over and over again. 'I should be in hospital.' Karen, the home manager, was happy to support Bob in his decision, but worried about how cancer could be explained simply and how the support workers would cope with any questions. She didn't know where to go for advice. The person responsible for inspecting residential care homes remembered hearing me speak at a conference and contacted me for help. I visited Lily's carers to give them some support, and Karen asked me question after question. How exactly could you explain cancer to someone with learning disabilities? What if Lily asked 'Take the cancer out'? Should Lily be told that she is going to die? I suggested keeping explanations simple, honest and to the point, focusing on what is happening in the here and now. Lily has a lump called cancer; it hurts; no, the doctors can't take it out. At this stage, don't tell her that she is going to die, unless she asks. In the future, you can build on this information by telling her that the cancer makes her tired and weak. Karen seemed happy with this advice: 'Yes, I see,' she said. 'We just need to tell her the truth.'

After Bob had told Lily that she had cancer, the support workers weren't sure how much Lily understood, but they felt that she certainly knew things were very serious. She was sad, tearful on one occasion. After Lily's death, Bob reflected on her understanding.

> 'I told her that she just had a little bit of cancer in her stomach. I said that's why she was in hospital. I called it "hospital", I never said "hospice". And she is not daft. She knows about cancer. Her dad died of it, and two aunties died of it. So I am sure that she would have understood about cancer. But she never asked, and that to me proves that she *did* understand. If she didn't understand, she would have asked me... If she really wanted to know something important, she *would* ask. I know she was disabled, but in some ways she was very mature... I think her way of coping with things was just not thinking about it. If she didn't want to know, she put the blinkers on. Out of sight, out of mind.'

It was difficult for me to gauge what Lily's understanding of her cancer was. I did not know her well enough to understand easily what she was saying, and as the weeks went by, she became too ill to talk, or maybe she simply lacked the inclination to do so. I had the following conversation with her after she was admitted to the hospice.

> *'Lily, do you know what is wrong with you?' 'Cancer. Stomach.' She gestures at her abdomen, which looks slightly swollen. 'You have cancer?' I ask. 'What is that? What is cancer?' 'Stomach.' 'What is it doing in your stomach?'*

'Eating.' 'Eating? The cancer is eating?' 'Yes.' 'What is it eating?' 'Everything. Haggis.' I am not sure whether Lily has understood my question, and whether she does indeed mean that the cancer is eating, or whether she heard 'stomach' and 'what is it eating', and is now telling me what she herself eats. I ask her again what cancer is. 'I don't know,' she says.

May, Bob's wife, wondered whether Lily knew more than everyone thought. In the weeks before she died, doctors at the hospice would stand around Lily's bed discussing her situation. Lily had her eyes closed, but May said, 'I am sure she can hear it all, but she would never talk about it.'

Karen and her staff had concerns about the other residents in the home, who had not been told the diagnosis or the outlook. The residents did not make too many demands on the support workers, and seemed to understand that Lily needed attention. Nobody had asked any questions, but the staff agreed that they must have been wondering what was going on. They overheard telephone conversations. They were asked not to bother Lily, to give her some privacy. The staff were at a loss about how to support them. Should they be told? What was best? Would it be damaging if they were kept away from things? They might be imagining all sorts of things. And in the end, they would know anyway, because Lily would die.

Once they realised what was wrong with Lily, her peers made no attempts to be tactful. One day, she was visited in the hospice by a house mate who asked Lily what was wrong with her. Lily answered that she had cancer in her tummy. 'Cancer,' the house mate said, 'that's what people die of.' Lily looked away, as if she hadn't heard or hadn't wanted to respond.

The support workers themselves also struggled with a lack of understanding. 'The doctors keep telling us about lesions,' said Karen. 'What *are* these lesions?' She hadn't realised that 'lesions' was, in this case, the word doctors used for 'cancer'.

Were people told the truth?

Eleven of the 13 men and women were told that they had cancer. However, only two of them asked their doctors further questions and were helped to understand the implications of their diagnosis. Four people lacked the verbal ability to express understanding or to ask questions; all the others either had unanswered questions, or did not ask.

The decision not to tell, or not to give further explanations, was sometimes taken by family and social care staff in the belief that this would protect the person from worry and distress. Some people were deliberately protected from understanding the truth, even when they asked.

Being told by a doctor

Most patients in the general population will be told of their cancer diagnosis by a doctor. In the Veronica Project, only John Davies, Vincent Sweeney and Amanda Cresswell were told by a doctor at the time of diagnosis. This may be because they had good verbal ability and had reached a degree of independence. They sometimes saw doctors on their own, without a relative or carer to support them.

Pete Carpenter was also told of his diagnosis by a doctor, but later and very reluctantly, and only at the insistence of social care staff who did not want to tell Pete themselves.

Vincent clearly grasped the severity of the situation when his doctor gave the diagnosis. 'I couldn't take it,' he said. 'I had to go out... I was crying and crying.' Seeing his sister-in-law cry confirmed for him how bad it was. However, Vincent found it very difficult to take in the full implications of cancer. His sister-in-law said:

> 'He doesn't know he is going to die. Or I don't think he does. We haven't told him. He knows he's got cancer, and maybe deep down he knows, because the doctors did say to him there's no cure, but the penny doesn't seem to have dropped. He gets depressed. I suppose at some point he has to be told.'

Vincent seemed confused about his cancer and the prognosis – and who could blame him? His doctor had once said that he wouldn't live to see Christmas, but he celebrated not only that Christmas, but the following Christmas as well, with no signs of serious decline. He had worrying questions in his mind, and it was never very clear whether he really wanted to know the answers. Once, I asked him whether he understood what cancer was.

> *I explain that some people know about cancer, maybe because they have seen it in someone else in their family, and some people don't understand it at all. Did anyone explain it to him? 'No,' he says. Would he like to know? 'Go on then,' he says, smiling at me, as if daring me.*
>
> *I don't comply immediately. I tell him there are all sorts of cancer, and I don't know any more about his particular cancer than he does. But I could explain cancer in general. I ask him first what cancer means to him, what he understands. 'Well, I know there are different kinds,' he says. 'I know someone who has got breast cancer, and that's different again, isn't it?'*
>
> *Shall I explain it to him? I ask him this question again. This time, he answers differently. 'No, don't,' he says. 'I would only worry about it. I would be sitting here after you've gone, and think about everything you have said, and it would go round and round in my head.'*

There were occasional hints that Vincent realised he was terminally ill. Four months after I met him he suddenly asked me, 'When is that book coming out? Am I going to be around to see it?' I told him truthfully that I really didn't know; it would be a couple of years from now.[8]

Only John and Amanda demonstrated a clear and full understanding of their cancer and its implications; both asked their doctors detailed questions.

Telling Amanda Cresswell what was wrong with her

Amanda's most vivid memories of her cancer were about information and disclosure. Not knowing what was happening when she was first admitted to hospital for investigations was one of the most frightening aspects of her illness.

> 'They did a quite a few tests, but they still weren't 100 per cent sure what was going on. I spent the whole night in casualty, and nobody was telling me what was going on apart from this one nurse who was really, really nice. She came in and was checking on me every five minutes, and she asked me whether I knew what was going on. I said, "I'm sorry, I still don't know what is going on." The nurse got really annoyed with one of

> the doctors. She said, "Look, this person has got a learning disability, she's left on her own, she's scared," and the nurse stayed with me then. I didn't like that hospital. They talked to me, but they were using language that I didn't understand, and I was saying, "Can you say it in an easier way?" but I don't think they really understood how I was really feeling. I was crying, I was feeling really down and depressed. I didn't have a clue what was going on and I was very, very scared. So I was glad when they transferred me to another hospital after three or four days. But it was also very frightening, because they didn't tell me what was wrong with me. All they said was, "We're transferring you because they've got better facilities in that hospital."'

She then explained what happened when the consultant in the next hospital told her about her cancer.

> 'It was a bit scary, because at the time my carers hadn't arrived to this hospital yet. Nobody had told them that I was transferred to another hospital. And then the doctor told me on my own what was wrong with me. He came and he introduced himself, and he asked me did I know what was wrong with me, and I said, "No, I don't know, the other hospital didn't tell me what was wrong." And then he said to me, "You've got non-Hodgkin's lymphoma." And I said to him, "What is that?" and then he said to me, "It's cancer in your lymph glands."'

At the time of her diagnosis, Amanda, who was an actress with a theatre company, happened to be working on a play to help people with learning disabilities understand issues about cancer. One of the messages of this play had been: 'If you don't understand what the doctor is saying, ask.' Amanda had been empowered by this. It helped her to be assertive with her doctor and ask what lymphoma was. She continued:

> 'I was *very* shocked, and then he was asking me, "Who do you live with?", and things like this. I had a phone in my room, and then my carer phoned me and he said do I know what's wrong with me yet. I said, "Yes, this is something, I am going to tell you, but I cannot tell you over the phone," and then they said, "Right, we're going to come and visit you, is there anything

> you need?" I said to him, "Please bring the bible," because I wanted to pray. Then he passed me to his wife and she said, "Amanda, are you OK?" I nearly started crying, I said, "I can't tell you over the phone." Then they spoke to a doctor, and then the doctor wouldn't tell them because I said, "Please no, don't tell them, this is something I have to do myself, it cannot be done over the phone." When they came, I just burst into tears. I took a few minutes – I had a big glass of water, and then I told them what was wrong. I just felt that I had to do that myself – that was something I *had* to do myself, definitely. And I'm glad I did.
>
> I didn't know what lymphoma was until they explained it to me. The doctor explained to me that there was a tumour growing inside my lymph glands. My doctor is fantastic, he is very very nice, and he said it's nothing that I've done wrong – any young person can get it, and they don't understand *why* you get it. I told him that my mum died of a brain tumour, and I asked him, "Is it hereditary?" He said, "Sometimes if somebody has had cancer, not in all families, but in some families you are likely to be exposed to it." Well, so, I'm just lucky that he got it in time. My biggest shock was that this tumour was growing inside of me, and I didn't even know it was growing inside of me. Especially when he showed me how big it was on the X-ray. It was the size of a football. And the reason I couldn't eat properly was because it was pressing right up inside me.'

What is striking is the level of Amanda's anxiety and fear, despite the fact that she was a strong self-advocate who took the initiative to ask questions whenever she was unsure.

Amanda's insistence on telling her foster carers herself that she has cancer may well have stemmed from a traumatic earlier experience of not being told that her mother had cancer. Amanda's life had been full of difficulties. She was born with brain damage, leading to mild cerebral palsy and learning disabilities. When she was a baby, her father was killed in a car crash. She lived with an aunt until her mother recovered from the injuries sustained in that crash. Amanda was bullied at school. Her mother, whom she was very close to, died of a brain tumour when she was 14. She was physically and financially abused by a foster carer when she was in her early twenties. Her diagnosis of lymphoma came at the age of 30, and she went through an aggressive programme of treatments. When I asked Amanda what the most difficult time in her life had been, she said without a moment's hesitation:

> 'That my mum didn't tell me that she was sick. I still regret it now. She never told me that she was dying... She wanted to protect me. Of course, things like that are upsetting, but it's definitely better to know. She used to be in a bad mood all the time, she used to shout at me, it was horrible. And of course I didn't understand why!'

Being told by family and carers

Most of the people needed paid carers or relatives to support them in their daily lives, and these supporters were always told first. It was left to them to decide whether, and how, to tell their client or relative. Families and social care staff struggled with the challenges this brought. They worried intensely about truth-telling and communication. They had no training or experience in breaking bad news, and their inclination was to protect the person with learning disabilities from distress as much as possible. They found it particularly difficult to talk about death and dying.

There was little or no support for these carers from outside professionals. Medical staff did not help families and social care staff in breaking bad news, and neither did they challenge protection from the truth. Most medical staff thought that the person's closest carers knew best, and left it at that.

Pete Carpenter had severe learning disabilities and lived in a staffed residential care home. When his carers were told that Pete had lung cancer and only had a few months left to live, they felt that it was important he was told his diagnosis. Others at Pete's day centre were beginning to speculate about cancer. 'I don't have cancer, I'm not dying like Pete, it's his own fault for smoking so much,' one woman said, even before Pete's cancer diagnosis. The staff wanted to be open. They thought that he would be able to understand what cancer was, particularly as his father had died of cancer when he was younger. However, they felt unable to break the bad news themselves; they believed that this was a doctor's task, although they were happy to support and reinforce the message. It proved very difficult to find a member of the medical team willing to do this. The hospital consultant wrote in a letter to the GP:

> 'I did try to explore with Mr Carpenter today his understanding with respect to his current illness. He is extremely well supported by his care workers who have explained to him that he is very ill and not going to get better. It was not really possible today to get much beyond this as Pete was easily preoccupied with a magazine... I did explain to him that tests so far have shown a serious problem but it did not seem appropriate to go further as he did not wish to hear any further news. I suspect that this is something that will need to be explored gradually with him over time, and may be better delivered in his own environment.'

Despite the support workers' clear requests that the doctors tell Pete that he had cancer, the doctors felt that they shouldn't tell him. The support workers explained to the doctors that Pete was unlikely to respond verbally to any probing about his insight or wishes. When a general practitioner finally told Pete that he had cancer, Pete didn't seem to grasp what was being said. However, his support workers now felt that they could explain to him why he was getting so tired and breathless. Pete seemed to understand a little more each time and did not show any signs of distress at being told.

Ben Edwards had severe learning disabilities and limited speech, although his verbal understanding was good. He had cancer in an undescended testicle, and had simply been told by Yanna, his home manager, that there was 'a lump in his tummy'. Yanna talked of her shock when Ben suddenly told her one day, 'I am dying.' He was in hospital for an operation and was physically very unwell at the time. Yanna remembered:

> 'I was mortified. Because it came completely out of the blue. I wasn't expecting it. I said to him, "No, you're not dying." But then I was talking to someone afterwards, and they said that I shouldn't have said that. So I went back to Ben a few more times to talk about it. Because he said it a couple more times after that, "I am dying, I am dying." I said to him then: "Nobody knows when any of us is going to die."'

When I give talks and training sessions about end-of-life care for people with learning disabilities, 'What do we say?' and 'How do we say it?' are among the most frequently asked questions. Families and non-medical carers often don't know what language to use when talking about cancer or dying to a person with learning disabilities. Those who want to tell the truth sometimes make it far too complicated, and can be put off by their own knowledge of the complexities of cancer, wondering how on earth they can explain it all. One support worker (unconnected to the Veronica Project) needed to explain chemotherapy to a woman with learning disabilities whose grasp of abstract concepts was poor. This support worker had tried to explain not only what cancer was and how the treatment would work, but also what the chances were of the chemotherapy being successful. She had used the image of people on a bus, explaining that 'if all these people on the bus would have the treatment, it would work for this many and not work for that many,' leaving the woman mystified. The truth is often not complicated, and can be told fairly simply. I advised her to explain no more than that the chemotherapy is a medicine, that it comes in a drip, and that the doctors hope that it will take the cancer away – but they can't be sure that it will; they just want to try.

Not being told

There was a sense among learning disability staff, particularly those supporting people with moderate, severe or profound learning disabilities, that it was better for the person not to know, as this protected them from anxiety and worry.

Sometimes, a decision not to inform the person with learning disabilities was founded on support workers' own attitudes around truth-telling. Mary, Nick Ballard's home manager, said: 'Nick doesn't know he has cancer. I think it is much better that way. He is quite happy, he just carries on. If it was me, I wouldn't want to know. He doesn't worry.'

One of the support workers for Marion Prentice thought:

> 'What is the point of putting people through worry, and add stress? Why would she need more tests? They are talking about a scan, but why? Because it is what *we* want to know. There is no point for *her* in knowing.'

A failure to explain the meaning of cancer does not always indicate a deliberate withholding of the truth. The concept of cancer may simply be too complex for some people with severe or profound learning disabilities. Yanna, the home manager for Ben Edwards, said:

> 'I don't think he really understands. I have told him that there is a lump in his tummy and that it shouldn't be there, and that the doctors had to take it out. He seemed to be happy with that. And with the radiotherapy, I tell him it is like photos. Because he doesn't understand what radiotherapy is, there is no way he could understand that. He is fine, lying down for it. Sometimes he calls for me, but I am always in the room when he is having it done.'

Yanna explained that Ben was always present in the consulting room when the cancer was discussed. 'But it goes over his head, really. He doesn't understand it.' Yanna was thus left with the task of explaining things to Ben afterwards. She didn't find this too difficult, although she described herself as 'no expert'. 'I don't make it too complicated,' she said. 'I keep it really simple. I think that's enough.' She added:

> 'I am absolutely convinced that Ben is the way he is now, because he doesn't worry. He is not like all the other people in the waiting room who are sitting there worrying about what the doctor is going to say, and what is going to happen to them. He is just worrying that it is taking too long and he can't get to his videos and his lunch in time.'

Some people don't want to know

When people don't want to know what is happening, they may well employ effective strategies to block out the truth. 'Denial' can be a successful coping strategy, and it is important to be sensitive to this need. When Ursula Smith was first told about her diagnosis of breast cancer years ago, she seemed to understand and accept this. She had a lumpectomy and radiotherapy. However, when a recurrence of the cancer was found in her bones 14 years later, she vehemently denied that this was so. 'No I haven't,' she replied when her home manager said she had cancer. 'No cancer. Diabetes.' Ursula did indeed have diabetes as well, and she preferred to think that this was why she needed so many hospital appointments. She may well have been affected by the death of cancer of Nick Ballard in the same home, six months earlier.

Jenny, one of the house mates of Pete Carpenter, was very clear about her need not to think about cancer. When she was told that Pete had cancer she said, 'I don't want to know. I want happiness.' The home manager respected her wishes and did not press any further information on her.

The fear of distress

Whilst carers may have withheld the truth because they genuinely believed it was in people's best interest 'not to upset them', I sometimes wondered whether it was partly motivated by an unspoken fear of the possible distress of people with learning disabilities. Being with someone in distress is never easy, and facing distressing issues around cancer and dying may well be too difficult for carers themselves. Families, social care staff and health care staff all steered away from causing any possible distress. Perhaps they had a sense of insecurity about their own ability to cope with unknown emotions or unknown expressions of emotion, and the way such emotions might be contained or supported. There was often a kind of 'forced jollity' when the person with learning disabilities was in the room.

I have not found any evidence, either in the research I have read or the stories other people have told me over the years, that people with learning disabilities are less able to cope with bad news than the rest of the population. There was certainly no evidence of it in the Veronica Project. Some people didn't demonstrate feelings of distress when they were told of their cancer, and surprised those around them by remaining outwardly calm despite the undeniable evidence of their failing bodies. Others expressed extreme sadness, fear or worry. John Davies 'cried enough tears to fill a river'. Vincent Sweeney 'couldn't take it'. Such distress is by no means unusual, and to avoid it could be an infringement of people's right to the truth and amount to inequitable treatment. There can be few other vulnerable groups of adults in society who are as protected from the truth about cancer and dying as people with learning disabilities, simply because of a fear that it will cause distress.

Understanding cancer and dying

Whether or not people understood about their cancer, and (if they were dying) about their impending death, depended on the degree of their learning disability, as well as on how much they were told and helped to understand. The third major influence was the impact of their life experience.

The impact of life experience

Some people with very limited cognitive skills may understand because of their own concrete experience, whereas others, apparently more able, may find it very hard to take in diagnostic information. We cannot assume that those with poorer cognitive ability will inevitably have a poorer understanding. Linda McEnhill gives some poignant examples illustrating the importance of people's life experience.

> Dale [a respondent in a pilot study on breaking bad news to people with learning disabilities], living with and caring for his remaining terminally ill parent, told me in response to the question 'What is cancer?' that he had learned about it at school and that it was 'a disease that grows in your body, in your lungs and other places.' When I asked him whether it is a serious illness he said, 'Yes, very serious' but when I asked him whether he had then expected that his father would die of the disease, he said 'No I never expected that, no one told me.' Now faced with his mother's illness I asked him what he had thought when he had been told that she had cancer. He said 'I just froze, I thought, I am going to be on my own.' (McEnhill 2008, pp.160–161)

Most people in the Veronica Project had experienced a close relative's death of cancer, and this clearly affected the way they understood their diagnosis. Whilst some compared their own illness to that of a relative who had died of cancer, wondering whether or not the outcome would be the same for them; others lacked insight into the subtleties and different possible outcomes of cancer.

Sally Burnett's father had cancer 12 years ago and died just a few months later. Her stepmother Joy kept telling Sally that her cancer was different; unlike her father, she was 'living with cancer'.

The experience of his father's death, combined with his own physical decline, helped Richard Horwood to understand what was happening to him. Richard had mild learning disabilities and was diagnosed with lung cancer that couldn't be cured. When I first met Richard, he told me how his father had died 13 years ago: 'He had lung cancer. Same as me. He died of it... I've got a little bit of cancer. That's not going to go away. It's only small. I won't die of it.' A few months later, Richard's physical deterioration set him thinking and worrying.

> 'It's got a little bit bigger. I am quite worried, actually. I am losing weight. That's what cancer does to you. When I was weighed before, I was 12 stone and 8 pounds. Now I am down to 11 stone and 1 pound. My father, when he had cancer he went down to 7 stone.'

When I paid Richard a follow-up visit two years later, he was much clearer about his prognosis. He had requested to move from his own flat into a nursing home, because of his increased support needs.

> *I ask, 'Do you think you'll get stronger again?' 'No, I don't think so,' Richard says. 'Cancer never goes away. It makes you weaker. It happened to my dad, he died of cancer, he didn't get stronger. He got weaker and weaker and then suddenly he died.' He tells me this matter-of-factly. I pause before asking him in an ordinary, interested tone of voice: 'Do you think that will happen to you, too?' 'Yes, I think it might,' Richard answers immediately. 'I think it will. Because that is what happens. I don't dwell on it.'*

Living and dying at the same time

It is not unusual for patients to live with the knowledge of approaching death, yet block that knowledge out for much of the time in order to cope with daily living. It is unkind, even cruel, to make someone focus on the truth of dying at all times. People can be 'living and dying' at the same time.

John Davies demonstrated this. The week he discovered that his cancer had returned, he said:

> 'I texted my friends last night. I said, "The cancer is back and I'm going to have chemotherapy and it's going to be all right,"

> and they rang me and went "Oh dear oh dear." I said, "Don't give me any oh dears, I've done my crying, I've cried lots but now that's done, I am going to get on with this. I am going to get on top of it. So sod off with your oh dear. I am going to be home for Christmas, I am going to sit down at my mum's – and her Christmas dinners! Ahhh... She makes her own stuffing, it's lovely. So that's all right, isn't it. What are you going oh dear for? It's all right. And then the chemo will get rid of this bit of cancer and it will be all right."'

Such upbeat behaviour could easily be mistaken for a lack of understanding and insight. Indeed, I wondered how much John had actually been told by his doctors. However, during an in-depth interview the following day, John demonstrated full understanding of his condition. 'It's coming up to Christmas, and that's my favourite time, being with friends and family. And they're going to make it special. Because of me being in hospital, you know?' He stopped, then continued speaking slowly, with long pauses. 'I think they think...well, they think the same as me. They've not said it, but... See, I think...that I'm dying. And they know that. My mum's not said it.'

During the following months, John remained openly optimistic whilst also regularly hinting at his knowledge that he would die soon. He was 'living and dying with cancer'. His outward optimism may be partly attributed to the needs of those around him not to talk about painful truths, and partly to his own need for keeping up hope; it certainly wasn't due to an inability to understand.

But the initial blocking out of the truth by cancer patients may well make way for a need to know and understand more. It can be a delicate balancing act to break bad news yet not take away hope, and to support the patient with an appropriate level of information throughout his or her illness. Usually, doctors and nurses can take their cue from the patient. The difference for people with learning disabilities is that they often need a lot more help to understand what is happening to them; they depend on others to give them information in a way they can understand, and they often need help to make sense of the information.

Increasing weakness helped people to understand

Even people who were not told, or who didn't talk about their cancer, seemed to work out eventually that they were dying, as their failing bodies made it clear. A few weeks before she died Sally Burnett said, 'I am dying.' She had never been told that her cancer was terminal. Two days before he died John Davies said, 'I am on my way to heaven.'

It was difficult to know with certainty how much people with more severe cognitive impairments understood, but most people who died seemed to accept their final deterioration calmly and with grace.

Ursula Smith had no family and was closely attached to Mary, her home manager. She was admitted to hospital two days before she died, and was highly distressed for much of the time. She begged Mary to take her home. Mary reflected the day after Ursula's death:

> 'The strange thing was, at lunchtime yesterday she actually sent me away. She would never touch you. If you touched her hand, she would push you away. But after she had her lunch yesterday, she stroked my face, and held my chin, and she gripped my hand really tight. And she said, "You can go now."'

Mary left for a few hours, and when she came back Ursula had become drowsy. She died in the evening.

Is ignorance bliss?

Social care staff and relatives often expressed the view that 'ignorance is bliss'. People who don't know cannot worry. This seemed to be mostly true for those people with severe and profound learning disabilities who genuinely lacked capacity to understand the implications of their illness. Their ability to live in the present moment protected them from the harmful effects of worrying. Ben Edwards' brother explained:

> 'He just keeps going. I really don't think he is worried in his mind. He is very matter-of-fact. I've got a pain, go to the doctor, yes, good idea, end of story. He doesn't seem to question the ins and outs. It's marvellous, really. I think we could all learn from that.'

People in the general population who face terminal illness are often heard to say that in order to cope, they had to learn to 'take each day as it comes'. Many people with learning disabilities, particularly those with more severe disabilities, already have the skill of 'taking each day as it comes', and this may explain some of their resilience when faced with a life-limiting illness.

The statement that 'ignorance is bliss' did not, however, seem to be true for those who *could* be helped to understand. On the contrary: some people were clearly distressed about not being given enough information to understand what was happening. Half understanding could be worse than full understanding.

Sally Burnett: 'Don't tell her'

Sally Burnett was not told the truth about her cancer and dying until her final weeks. Her story shows not only the ways in which Sally's family and the hospice staff prevented her from understanding, but also their motivations, and the effect that this protection from the truth had on Sally.

Sally was 45 years old. She had autism and mild learning disabilities. Sally was a slight woman who, at first impressions, seemed rather vulnerable; but she knew what she wanted and was very determined. She had overcome childhood predictions that she would never amount to much, eventually competing in national athletics contests. The wall of her room was lined with medals. She loved to dance, always the first on the dance floor and the last to leave. Her social worker helped her to find a job stacking shelves in the local supermarket for a couple of hours each week. Sally was not naturally sociable and found it difficult to maintain conversations – being hard of hearing didn't help. She tended to answer questions briefly, in a booming, monotonous voice.

Sally's father was diagnosed with cancer 12 years ago. His illness was short; he died within a couple of months. Sally knew he had cancer, and she knew that it had caused his death. She lived with her stepmother Joy for another couple of years whilst preparing to move into her own flat. She was proud of her new-found independence, and loved having a place of her own. She relied on Joy for day-to-day support, who telephoned every day and visited several times a week. Joy had been in Sally's life since she was a young child, and quickly became like a mother to her. Sally called her 'Mum'.

Despite the many things she enjoyed, life had not been altogether easy for Sally. She used to poke herself in the eye with her fist, or throw things. Joy had worked hard at helping her to stop this. 'I said to her, if you're feeling like that, just clap your hands instead, and sing! Just sing out everything that's inside. You can sing "I'm having a bad day and I'm fed up!"'

Sally had not injured herself for many years now. Her social worker was impressed with how well she coped with life. 'She is very together, very feisty.'

Sally remembered how cancer of her bowel was diagnosed five years ago. 'I couldn't go toilet from my bottom. I rang me mum and told her.' She also explained what had happened when Joy took her to the doctor: 'Professor did an operation. Gave me a bag. It goes in the bag now.' She learned how to cope with her colostomy bag[9] independently.

When she was diagnosed with cancer, Sally immediately made the connection with her father's death. She asked Joy repeatedly, 'Am I going to die? Is this going to kill me, Mum?' Throughout the following years, Joy kept explaining that her cancer was not the same as her dad's, that this could be treated, and although 'any cancer can kill you', she was lucky to have had those treatments. It would never go away completely, but she would now be 'living with cancer'. Joy was deeply worried that if Sally were told that her illness was terminal, she would at best get depressed, and at worst start hurting herself again. 'She would just give up,' said Joy. 'She would just cry and cry. She would be so upset.' What was the point of Sally knowing the truth? Sally appeared content with Joy's explanations. When I asked Joy why she thought Sally asked if she was going to die, she answered, 'I think it is just something that she thought of. Her dad had cancer, and he died. So she thought: cancer, died. Everything is black and white with her. She doesn't understand things in-between very well.'

When I first met Sally, she had begun to feel the effects of advancing cancer. She was becoming more tired and had to give up work. She still attended her dance class most weeks, but this was also becoming more difficult to keep up. She missed her activities and her routines.

One day, Sally's legs suddenly swelled up and she was unable to pass urine. She was taken into hospital urgently and her family was told to prepare for the worst. Tests revealed that the cancer had grown and was now blocking her urethra, making it impossible to give her a urinary catheter. Instead, she was given a supra-pubic catheter[10] and she rallied. I visited her a few days later, finding her looking very frail. She understood what had happened in the most practical terms, telling me simply about her symptoms and their effect.

> *'You are in hospital,' I say. She nods. 'What has been happening?' I ask. 'I've been sick.' What, I mime, sick? Yes, she nods. I sit with her for a while, not saying much. I hold her hand. After a few minutes, she says, 'I came in on Friday.' 'You came in on Friday,' I repeat. 'With your mum?' 'Yes. Water wouldn't come out.' Pause. 'Water wouldn't come out?' I ask. 'Oh dear. Did it hurt?' 'Yes, it did hurt.' Pause. 'I got a tube.' Then, 'They couldn't get a tube in.'*
>
> *After a while I ask, 'Did your legs get big?' She nods (and throughout my visit, she mostly nods, and sometimes shakes her head, in simple answer to questions from medical staff). She adds, 'My legs were all swollen.' 'Oh dear,' I say again. 'That must have been uncomfortable. Where they really heavy?' 'Yes,' she says. 'I couldn't stand.'*

Sally was referred to the hospital palliative care team, and a sensitive nurse met with Joy, acknowledging that Sally was now in the final stages of cancer, and suggesting a referral to the hospice. It was the only time during my involvement with this family that I saw Joy cry; she always came across as cheerful and competent. Joy was the archetypal carer; now retired, she spent her time looking after not only Sally but also assorted other relatives who needed care and support. She made people feel at ease, hugging me on our first meeting, patting my cheek, looking after me the way she looked after everyone else. It was her task to keep everyone informed, to encourage Sally's brothers to visit, to help Sally's aunts and uncles to relate to her. 'Tell Sally…' 'Sally, tell your aunt what you did…'

Joy explained to Sally that there were 'special hospitals for cancer, called hospices', and Sally was quite happy to be transferred. Joy took great pains to tell everyone that Sally must not be told the truth about her poor prognosis. This is what happened on Sally's first assessment by the hospice doctor.

> *The doctor and Joy have a discussion about Sally's insight, speaking softly, so Sally cannot hear them. The doctor asks, 'How much does Sally know?' 'She knows she has cancer. But that is all she knows. She asks sometimes, and I tell her that this is not the same as her father's cancer, that it can be treated. And it can, you know! They did treat it.' The doctor nods. Joy continues, 'As long as you are upbeat, she is quite happy. So if you could leave it at that, please, I would appreciate it. Just be positive, and reassure her.' The doctor does not challenge this... As Joy kisses her goodbye, Sally asks, 'Am I going to be all right?' 'Of course!' says Joy cheerfully. 'Everything will be all right. OK?' Sally nods, then stares ahead.*

Although Sally was initially helped to walk the length of the hospice corridor, this became increasingly difficult. When she was hardly able to stand up without support, it was clear to everyone that she would not be able to go back to her flat. Sally's desire to go back to her flat dominated my visits during the ensuing months. Sally didn't often initiate conversation, but when she did, it was usually to tell me that her legs were weak and that she missed her flat. Nobody acknowledged with her that she would never be able to go back. Joy told her that she could go back when she was stronger, and the hospice staff went along with this, cheerfully trying to make her do her exercises and build up strength. As a result, the physiotherapist became the most important staff member for Sally. As she tried moving her legs, Sally struggled with the realisation that all these exercises did not have the desired result.

Joy was aware of Sally's desperation. 'She is getting more tearful... She keeps saying: "Mum, I want to keep strong!" She really is weak now. She is not getting out of bed any more. She still wants to go back to her flat, and she knows she can't whilst she is so weak... So I tell her, "You will, love, don't you keep fretting about it. Your flat is still there, and when you're better you will go back to it."' Twice, Sally managed to go on a visit to her flat for just a couple of hours.

When Sally was first admitted to the hospice, she asked Joy again whether she was going to die. 'I squashed that right on the head,' said Joy. Sally never asked again. 'But if she did, I would give her the same answer. I would say, "We're all going to die one day, and you need to keep your strength up, and you'll be all right." I would never tell her "Yes, you are going to die."'

Sally became increasingly distressed. The following are extracts from my notes written during the two months before she died.

I can hear Sally crying as I walk into the room. She is not yet aware of my presence – she is crying alone. I walk to her bedside, she looks at me, briefly stops making the crying sound but doesn't smile, and soon starts crying again. I lean over, take her hand. 'Oh dear, Sally...' I say, taking a few seconds just to be with her. Then, 'What is it?' 'I can't walk,' she wails. 'I know you can't walk,' I say. 'It is sad. Does it make you feel sad?' She nods. 'Yes,' she says, and cries some more.

I stay with her for a few more seconds, just holding her hand. 'I am going to take my coat off, and get a chair, and sit down with you,' I say. By the time I am settled, the crying has stopped. She volunteers, 'I went to my flat on Monday.' 'I know! Your mum told me. What happened?' 'I went in the lift. I went to the first floor. I saw the dinner ladies. I went to see my neighbour. Only one was in.'

'What was it like?' I ask. 'To be in your flat? Was it good or bad? Good or sad?' I mime these last two statements: thumbs up, thumbs down. 'Good!' she gestures, and smiles. 'What was good about it?' I ask. 'What did you like about being in your flat?' 'Seeing my rooms. My bedroom. My bathroom.' 'Your sofa,' I add. 'Your kitchen corner.' She smiles. 'Yes.' 'What did you do when you were in your flat?' 'Had something to drink. Watch TV.'

I ask her whether she would like to go back to her flat again, or whether once was enough (I am learning to give her two alternatives, rather than ask a yes/no question, because of her tendency to answer 'yes' if she hasn't quite heard or understood). She is very clear: 'Go back again. I want to go for another visit to my flat.'

I feel comfortable, sitting here with Sally; maybe this is the first time I feel truly comfortable, without the need to ask questions simply to fill the empty space. The space is not empty. She is full; I am content and comfortable just to let her be, just to sit with her. The weeks spent getting to know her are beginning to pay off.

During the next hour, she begins to cry again many times. At least once every five or ten minutes. This is not simply a contortion of facial features, lasting a couple of seconds, over as soon as it begins: it is real crying. She sometimes stops fairly abruptly, but still looks distressed, staring ahead of her with a frown and deeply worried eyes; and will then either turn to me and talk (ranging from 'I can't move my legs' to 'How was your weekend?') or cry some more. Here is a woman in real distress. 'I can't walk,' she repeats each time. 'I can't move my legs.'

There is nothing I can say except acknowledge how hard that must be. I am leaning over the side bar of her bed, with my arms resting on the high mattress; and I either take her hand or have my hand close enough for her to take, which sometimes she does.

Her legs are twitching. At first I think that she has restless legs, but then I realise that she is actually trying to move them, trying to do some exercises. She is very weak and shaky. 'I need the physio,' she cries. She wants to get stronger.

She asks for the bed sheets to be pulled off her legs, then pulled up again, then off again. Her legs are pale, smooth, puffy. Her short nightdress only just manages to cover her incontinence pad. There are frequent loud gurgling sounds from her colostomy bag.

We sit, we talk a bit, she sometimes looks at me and smiles, but most of the time she looks distraught, and she cries. And I sit with her, in turmoil at first. It is so very, very hard to sit with someone in such deep distress. This is not just a passing episode of tearfulness, I know. This is a deep suffering, borne of the knowledge that she is not getting stronger, that her strength (and possibly, by implication, her life – but I don't know how much she is conscious of this) is slowly slipping through her hands; that she cannot get a grip on it. And as far as I can see, there is no one – absolutely no one – who allows her to be distressed by this, to be sad; no one to help her come to terms with it. Everyone I have heard so far (family and staff alike) have jollied her along, telling her to try and get stronger, and I am in turmoil because I know (and everyone else must know) that she is only going to get weaker. Even the most vigorous exercises in the world will not get Sally her strength back. She is slowly dying. [...]

Sally rings the buzzer, and a nurse walks in. 'I can't move my legs,' Sally says. 'You are uncomfortable?' asks the nurse, apparently trying to repeat what Sally said. I help Sally out: 'She says that she can't move her legs.' 'I know that,' says the nurse. 'We know you can't move your legs.' And she sets about raising Sally's pillows, making her sit up a bit higher. 'She has also been asking for the physio,' I say. 'Yes, we don't know when she is coming,' says the nurse. 'The doctors haven't been yet either.' And she leaves.

Nurses leave. This is a revelation to me, having been in that role so often myself. As a nurse, I always thought I was present to my patients, but this nurse certainly wasn't. And I would probably have done exactly what she did. Cheerful, breezy, competent. What would I do now, if I walked in and my patient was crying, saying, 'I can't move my legs'? I hope I would sit down, take the patient's hand, and try to figure out exactly what she was saying. Why is that so distressing? What would she like? And what makes her cry?

Is the leg painful? Or does the consistent lack of movement indicate, with frightening clarity, that she is not getting better? Does she need painkillers, physiotherapy, or emotional and spiritual support?

[...] The physiotherapist comes in. 'I can't move my legs,' Sally says, almost crying again. The physio stays very cheerful. 'Don't say that! Come on.' She moves the bedclothes from Sally's legs: 'Go on, lift your legs up,' she says encouragingly. Sally does so, one by one, with some help from the physio. 'What do you mean, you can't move your legs! Look at you! That's wonderful!' breezes the physio.

A week later:

I ask Sally, 'How are you, really? How are you in your feelings?' 'All right,' she says. Then, after a brief pause: 'I still can't walk.' 'No,' I say. 'You have been thinking about that a lot, and it has been making you very sad.' She nods. She doesn't cry this time. Throughout this visit, she stares ahead of her with that pale, sad face.

I make one attempt at trying to find out what she really thinks. 'What would it be like,' I ask, 'if you did not get stronger? If you could never go back to your flat? What would that be like for you?' She shakes her head, looking away for a brief moment. Then she looks me in my eyes for what feels like a very long time, but what is probably no more than a minute. I have to tell myself explicitly not to look away, because that is the temptation; her gaze is steady and penetrating. She doesn't look away either; her eyes simply drift off mine, and she looks ahead of her again. Sad, sad, sad feelings in the air. Then, she picks up Hello magazine again and starts to leaf through it, reading some of it without looking at me. I wonder whether she is trying to shut me out, with my difficult questions. She has done that before, usually by closing her eyes as if she is going to sleep. I feel I cannot say any more. I cannot ask any more. She doesn't want to talk about it. We sit in silence. Once she has put the magazine back on the bedside table, we sit in silence.

[...] I have moved away from the bed, but when the nurse has gone, Sally suddenly starts crying and I go over again to take her hand. 'Oh dear, Sally...' 'I miss my flat,' she cries. 'My house.' 'Oh Sally,' is all I can say. 'It is so very hard for you, isn't it.' She nods.

Three weeks later:

We are silent for a long time. Sally doesn't close her eyes, but stares ahead of her, occasionally turning to me to smile. When I put my hand within reach, she unfolds her own and takes mine. Silence no longer feels uncomfortable. But it is not an easy silence. I look at Sally's face, and I glimpse a whole world behind her eyes, a deep sadness. This is what she does, day in day out, lying here, with only herself. It seems so incredibly lonely. I imagine her, even with her visitors, and I see her as isolated and lonely. Maybe she doesn't experience it as such; maybe she has been alone with herself all her life, and is used to it, maybe even likes it; but my interpretation of the world behind her resigned eyes is one of despair.

She breaks the silence herself. She turns to me and says, 'I have been here a long time.' I pause for a second, looking at her before replying, 'Yes, you have. Three months.' I hold up my fingers. 'That is a very long time.' She nods. Nothing more is said, so after a few minutes I make my usual attempt to talk more about this issue. 'Do you ever wonder whether you will get out of here at all?' I ask. She nods, but it is the nod she gives when she hasn't quite heard the question. She is very deaf. So I write it down on a pad of paper, and she reads out loud: 'You have been here a long time. I wonder if that makes you think sometimes: WILL I EVER GET OUT OF HERE?' She puts the pad down and looks ahead of her for a few seconds, then turns her face to me and nods slowly. Then she adds, 'I will when I get stronger.'

We don't speak any more about it. 'OK,' I say, and take her hand. It feels as if she knows that she can hint at such thoughts with me, but cannot bear to take it any further. Or maybe she really does believe that she will get strong enough to go home one day; maybe that is a hope she needs to hold on to so much that it is completely realistic to her. And it is, after all, what her mum tells her... I find it hard to leave her, because it feels so much as if I am leaving her abandoned in an impossibly painful world.

I struggled with the question whether the conspiracy of silence around Sally's imminent death, the forced jollity, caused her unnecessary distress. Was it ethical to withhold the truth from her? I understood Joy's reasons for not wanting to upset Sally, borne of a very close bond and a lifetime of genuine care and support; but I was somewhat troubled by the hospice staff's collusion with Joy, the lack of emotional support offered to either Joy or Sally. Having discussed it with my research advisory group, I raised the issue with the hospice team. The doctors, nurses and social worker said that Sally never indicated that she wondered about her future. The social worker explained:

'Her mum really knows her best, and understands everything about her learning disabilities, so I went with that... If Sally asked us such a straight question, like "Am I going to die?" or "Am I going to live at home again?", of course we would answer it. But she has never asked any of us. So we can't very well go in and talk to her about it.'

The hospice social worker talked to Joy a few times during the early weeks of admission, but after that, no family meetings were held, not with the social worker, not with the doctors, and not with the nurses. Joy sometimes caught up with staff in the corridor, but never asked to meet with them more formally. Sally was never seen by anyone whose explicit task it was to give her emotional support.

Later, I found very regular entries in the hospice notes saying that Sally was distressed, that she had been crying; but throughout her stay, the only action taken was to give her more physiotherapy. The cheerful physiotherapist would sing songs with her, encouraging her to walk, and often Sally responded; she would stop crying and sing along with a serious face, as if setting out on a long journey.

Sally's failing body eventually told her that she was dying, but she had to work out this truth for herself. When she was completely bed-bound and death was just weeks away, she spoke of her thoughts to those around her. Joy described how she then supported Sally:

> 'She said to me, "I think I'm dying, Mum." So I said to her, "Yes, well, we can't know for sure, there's always miracles, but I think it might be your time, love, like it was your father's time. And he was very peaceful, I think he was going to see your mum. We can't know that for sure but that's what I think will happen, so I think you will be OK, love, I think you'll be seeing your mum and dad." And she was quite peaceful after that.'

After Sally's death, I went back to the hospice to meet with the staff team. One of the nurses said:

> 'She *did* know. And she talked about it. It always took a long time with her. You had to stay with her for five, ten minutes before she would tell you something. Or ask you questions. It was about three weeks before she died, and I was with her, spending some time. And she said to me, "I am never going to walk again. It is not going to be long." She was fine when she said that. She was quite calm, really.'

A nursing assistant added, 'I think she did give up in the end, but she was very calm about it. She said to me, about a week before she died: "I am dying."'

When I was preparing this book and Joy read the first draft, she reflected:

> 'You know, reading what you wrote made me wonder whether I'd done the right thing. Should I have told Sally the truth when she asked me "Will I die?" But I still think it was right not to tell her. I know my Sally. Her autism was such that she would not have got past the answer, and every waking moment would be eaten up by it. She would be crying and self-harming about it. When she was given the colostomy bag, she was told that she couldn't have certain foods, like fizzy lemonade. She never drank fizzy lemonade much, but that upset her until the day she died. She'd be staring ahead of her, and I'd say, "What's up, Sally?" and she'd say, "Can't have lemonade." She self-harmed and cried during the night. So I think it was better that she didn't know. I still feel the best part of her cancer years were enriched with not knowing the full extent of the illness – and she carried on, in her way, with what she wanted to do.'

Joy's determination to protect Sally from worry, fear and distress was understandable. Her knowledge and understanding of Sally needed to be listened to and taken into account.

Families go through very difficult times: they are themselves trying to cope with the bad news, and are often devastated by it. Joy had to keep up hope for herself that Sally might one day come back home. To a lesser extent, this is also true for residential care staff who may have known their client for many years and are often deeply distressed by the cancer diagnosis.

While relatives and support staff of people with learning disabilities can be understandably protective, paternalistic attitudes may well be an infringement of patients' right to information. Studies of the general population have found that relatives' views on disclosure may not coincide with patients' views; even when patients want to know the truth, relatives are more inclined to keep it from them (Noone *et al.* 2000). It can be much more complex with patients who have learning disabilities, who may not be able to express their views on truth-telling. Carers may well have valid views that people should be protected from the profound distress caused by bad news; but this needs to be carefully balanced against people's need and right to know.

What was interesting about Sally's situation was the failure of hospice staff to help Sally understand what was happening, or to support Joy. Whilst Joy felt that she could always talk to the staff if she needed to, she did not ask them for meetings, and they did not offer. The strong feelings, emotions and opinions of families need to be acknowledged, but the needs of the patient must always come first. Rather than simply deferring to relatives and social care staff, medical staff should make their own assessment of the patient's need for information and discuss this with the carers, working with them and supporting them. Many people with learning disabilities don't ask questions, but that does not necessarily mean that they don't want to know what is happening. This may be challenging for health care staff, who often rely on spoken words when offering support.

Breaking bad news

What does 'truth-telling' mean?

Truth-telling is not simply a question of 'to tell or not to tell'. Some people with learning disabilities may be told that they have cancer, but that doesn't necessarily mean that they have understood what that means for them, or what the implications are. Others may not be told that they have cancer, but understand very clearly that their health is deteriorating, maybe even that they are dying. Truth-telling is not a one off event: it is a gradual process of helping someone discover and understand what is happening (Blackman and Todd 2005).

Telling cancer patients with learning disabilities 'you have cancer' is only the beginning of helping them to understand. There is so much more to explain. What is cancer? What does the patient understand about cancer? What is happening with this particular patient, and this particular cancer? What does the patient expect? What does the doctor expect? Are any cancer treatments being considered? Do choices have to be made? The full answers to all these questions may be too much to take in all at once, or too complex.

Truth-telling means, at its most basic, that everything we say is true – no lying. In practice, telling people with learning disabilities the truth about cancer includes any communication that is intended to help them understand what is happening. Sometimes, the words used by doctors, nurses, families and social care staff are not untrue, but if they are difficult words or medical jargon, used intentionally because the person will probably not understand them, they can become part of obscuring the truth. When Vincent Sweeney asked his doctor: 'It isn't going to kill me or anything?' his doctor answered truthfully that 'the tumour may well progress', but these words were unlikely to help Vincent realise the truth; they were probably chosen *because* they would prevent full understanding. Vincent did, indeed, believe that he had been given good news.

Attitudes to truth-telling

'Should we tell him about his diagnosis and prognosis, and if so, how?' These questions are not unique to families and carers of people with learning disabilities: they have also been a matter of much debate in the medical profession with regards to the general population. In western countries, there have been major shifts in attitude and practice. Before the 1970s, the vast majority of doctors did not tell cancer patients their diagnosis (Oken 1961), but studies carried out later found that almost all doctors now *did* tell their patients, and believed that this was better (Novack *et al.* 1971; Seale 1991). Seale (1991) found that most doctors and nurses preferred their patients to know that they were dying. Cancer patients themselves share this view, and are overwhelmingly in favour of openness and information (e.g. Jenkins, Fallowfield and Saul 2001; Leydon *et al.* 2000; Noone *et al.* 2000).

Much less is known about what happens when the patient has learning disabilities. There are only a few other studies that considered whether, and how, people with learning disabilities received information about a cancer diagnosis. These studies found that, unlike most people in the general population, they were often not told. The people with learning disabilities in those studies indicated that they wanted more information and openness about cancer and dying (McEnhill 2005; Todd 2004; Tuffrey-Wijne *et al.* 2007).

What is 'bad news'?

Vincent Sweeney was not alone in misunderstanding his doctor's ambiguous or incomplete information. One study found that only about half of a group of people in the general population understood that 'the tumour has progressed' was not good news (Chapman *et al.* 2003). A distinction clearly needs to be made between what the patient has been *told*, and what the patient has *understood*.

Bad news is 'any news that drastically and negatively alters the patient's view of her or his future' (Buckman 1984, p.1597). In other words, news is bad if you think that your future is less bright because of it. This means that the 'badness' of the news depends on the patient's sense of time and his or her ability to anticipate the future, requiring a level of abstract thinking that may be impaired in people with learning disabilities.

There are likely to be marked differences in this respect between people with mild or moderate learning disabilities and those with severe or profound learning disabilities. Some people with severe or profound learning disabilities lack the capacity to grasp the concept of 'future', and therefore may never realise that 'cancer' is bad news. In such cases, it is possible to talk freely about the person's cancer in his or her presence, without this being perceived as bad news. This was the case with Ben Edwards: he enjoyed sitting with Yanna and myself as we discussed his cancer, simply because he enjoyed being part of a conversation about himself.

Some people, on the other hand, may link the concept of cancer to that of dying, but lack the sense of time to put this into context. Their life experience may have taught them that, as Lily's house mate pointed out so clearly, 'Cancer is what you die of.' This is what worried Sally Burnett's stepmother Joy when she didn't tell Sally all those years ago that her cancer would kill her. She was truthful in telling Sally about her cancer and the necessary treatments, but she was careful not to 'drastically and negatively alter Sally's view of her future', trying hard not to make Sally see her cancer as 'bad news'. Was Joy being truthful, or was she withholding the truth? It could be that Joy's attempt to maintain that the cancer was not 'bad news' was actually more truthful to begin with. If Sally's poor sense of time meant that she would perceive death as being imminent, then telling her that her cancer would kill her would not be truthful. She had, after all, another five years of living to do. However, as time went by and it became clear that Sally *was* going to die within the next few months, the insistence that her cancer and the associated physical deterioration was not bad news ('You can go back to your flat when you're stronger') became untruthful.

Those for whom the distant future is too abstract may perceive 'bad news' as something very different from what we would expect. Ben Edwards' fellow patients in the waiting room probably worried about the possibility that the treatment might not work in the medium- to long-term future: that would be bad news. For Ben, 'bad news' was related to his immediate future: the possibility that he might miss lunch. For someone like Ben, who was unlikely to grasp the long-term implications of his cancer at this stage in his illness, 'breaking bad news' is more likely to involve regular explanations of the immediate future.

How to break bad news?

Nowadays, doctors and nurses are much better trained in breaking bad news than they were a few decades ago. Such training usually includes the recommendation to find out how much the patient already knows, and how much the patient *wants* to know. The information is then given in small chunks, including 'warning shots', such as 'I'm afraid the results of the test were not as good as we had hoped' (e.g. Baile *et al.* 2005; Girgis and Sanson-Fisher 1995; Ptacek and Eberhardt 1996).

Such guidelines are helpful, but it is not clear whether they work for all people with learning disabilities. For example, how can we assess the information preferences of someone who doesn't communicate in words, or who doesn't ask any questions?

Pete Carpenter was clearly unable to pick up his doctor's 'warning shots', as can be seen in the doctor's letter: 'I did explain to him that tests so far have shown a serious problem but it did not seem appropriate to go further as he did not wish to hear any further news.'

Vincent Sweeney was alarmed by one of his doctor's 'warning shots', panicking about its possible meaning, and not sure whether he had understood it. 'My doctor says that I should go and have a holiday whilst I still can. What is that supposed to mean? Whilst I still can?'

It is not always easy to know whether someone should be told the truth. The story of Sally Burnett shows how complex the considerations can be. There simply has not been enough research to show whether it is better for some people with learning disabilities not to tell them, and how we would be able to assess this. However, based on the experiences of the people in the Veronica Project, it seems that they coped well if those around them were open and honest, gave explanations in a simple way, and were warm and kind.

There may well be people for whom it is better if they don't know the full truth; but there should be explicit reasons for not telling the truth, and these should be made clear to everyone caring for the person. What seemed important for the people in the Veronica Project was that they were helped to understand as much as they possibly *could*, given their cognitive limitations, and as much as they *wanted* to. This did not happen for everyone. It was particularly difficult if decisions and responsibilities around disclosure rested with a single carer, without support from professionals and other carers.

Simple explanations

Amanda Cresswell pointed out most clearly that language needs to be simple, using non-ambiguous words that may sound blunt. She said:

> 'What doctors and nurses and other people should know is that it is really important people are told about their cancer. If they are not told, how can they understand it? They need to know! But they should tell people in a way that they can understand. They should say: "You've got something growing inside you, and we want to get rid of it, because if we don't, you are going to die."'

The willingness and ability to explain things simply is beneficial throughout someone's illness, not just when it comes to explaining the diagnosis. For some people, particularly those with severe or profound learning disabilities, simple explanations of day-to-day problems may well be all that is needed or appropriate. Yanna, Ben Edwards' support worker, managed this very well.

> *When Ben tells Yanna about his vomiting, he points to the kitchen. 'Don't blame my cooking!' laughs Jackie* [support worker]. *'Nobody else got sick.'*
>
> *'He always blames the food when he is sick,' Yanna tells me, and then turns to Ben: 'You were vomiting because your tummy is not well. We'll sort it out, love. I'll phone the doctor.'*

Summary

Whether or not to tell the people the truth about their illness was an issue for almost all carers.

Were people with learning disabilities told the truth about cancer and dying?

- Eleven out of 13 people were told that they had cancer, but only two understood the full implications.
- Most people were not helped to understand more about their illness.
- The few people who were given full and clear explanations found this very helpful. It enabled them to make treatment decisions and cope with the treatments.

Did people with learning disabilities understand cancer and dying?

- How much people understood depended on:
    - cognitive ability (some people with severe learning disabilities lacked the capacity to understand fully)
    - how much they were told and helped to understand
    - life experience (those who had lost a parent to cancer made the connection with their own prognosis).
- People can be 'living and dying at the same time': knowing the truth about approaching death, yet blocking out that

knowledge some of the time. This can be mistaken for a lack of understanding.

- Some people do not want to know the truth, or talk about it.
- Withholding the truth about dying could cause distress. One woman was confused by being told she would get better, and the conflicting evidence of her deteriorating health.
- Several people understood that they were dying, even if they weren't told, because their bodies were failing.

Breaking bad news

- Most people in the general population are told about their cancer and prognosis by a doctor. This was not the case for the people in the Veronica Project; only a few people with mild learning disabilities were told by their doctor.
- Families or support workers were usually told first about the diagnosis and prognosis. It was left up to them to tell their client or relative, or not. They found this difficult, lacking skills and confidence.
- Carers were not given any professional support in breaking bad news.
- Several people were completely protected from the truth.
- The decision whether or not to tell the truth was influenced by carers' personal attitudes. There was a sense among support workers and families that it was better not to tell because it would protect the person from worrying and getting upset.
- People should only be told as much as they want to know; but how much they want to know can be difficult to assess.
- Using language that is difficult to understand can be a way of obscuring the truth.
- Information should be clear, simple and to the point.

CHAPTER 4

Family and Friends

In several of the stories so far, families were prominent. More than the physical surroundings of home, hospital or hospice, more than the treatments, the activities and the outings, what mattered were the people sharing in it. John Davies and Vincent Sweeney longed to be with their families when they were very ill, despite their long struggle for independence. For Nick Ballard, the absence of family was poignant.

For many people in the Veronica Project, it was paid carers who provided most of the day-to-day support, and sometimes these seemed to be the only crucial people in their lives. However, as the study progressed, it became increasingly clear how much families mattered. This chapter looks at their place in people's stories, as well as the place of friends and peers.

Lily Lamb and her family

Lily grew up in the family home, together with her brother Bob who was two years older. Apart from a traumatic few years in her early teens, when she was sent to a boarding school for children with special needs, she lived with her parents. Lily's parents were caring and protective, 'over-protective' in Bob's eyes. They did everything for Lily, and she demanded it of them. She had a strong emotional bond with her mother, whom she followed around everywhere; she would even sit on a chair outside the toilet, waiting for her mother to emerge. When Bob brought May home, Lily threw a tantrum whilst her mother desperately tried to make a good impression on her son's new girlfriend. Bob thought that his parents shielded him from worrying about Lily. Even when their father was very old and Lily had gone to live in a residential care home, he insisted on going to Lily's annual appraisal meetings. Bob explained, 'I said I could go because I could see it was too much for him, but he didn't really want me to. It was as if he thought that Lily was his responsibility and shouldn't be mine.'

Lily's mother died suddenly of a heart attack. Lily was with her at the time and called her father, but it was already too late. Lily was, at that stage, on the waiting list to move into a residential home, but her father didn't want Lily to lose her family home at the same time as losing her mother, so they lived together for another decade. To everyone's surprise, Lily seemed to cope well with the loss of the mother she had been so exclusively focused on. She was composed at the funeral, shaking everyone's hand. When it was over she asked her father, 'What will happen to me now?' What happened was that she simply transferred her focus onto him.

He tried to do his very best for her. When he became old and frail, and Lily finally moved into the residential care home that her parents had originally chosen, she continued to visit him every other weekend. Her support worker at the home remembered:

> 'She wanted to go every weekend but we wanted to think of him too. It was hard for him in the end, because she was so much in control. She would have a plan for the whole weekend, and just tell him, "We are going to go here and there." And he would just drive her wherever she said. They would do the shopping for the weekend on the Friday night, with her pushing the trolley around the supermarket. She loved driving. Her father would drive her. They liked to go out into the countryside, just to have a look. She always liked that, even when she was with us. She loves driving out in the minibus. And if she has a choice, she would demand to go to a country estate or something like that. Not that she is very active physically, she just liked to sit and look around. Like she did with her dad.'

When Lily's father was in his late eighties he was diagnosed with cancer. He died only two weeks later. Again, Lily surprised everyone by coping well; her support workers had expected her to be devastated and to become depressed. This time, she transferred her attention to her brother Bob, and he became the person she wanted to be with, the only person she would tell what was worrying her, the person she would ask questions if she wanted to understand something. However, I caught glimpses of an ongoing presence of her father in her mind.

> *She asks about my children. I cannot quite understand whether she asks how many or how young, so I get a photograph out of my Filofax and show it to her. She looks at it, then asks, 'Have they got a dad?' I say, 'Yes, he is my husband,' but she persists, pointing at my children in the photograph: 'No, THEY, have THEY got a dad?' I make it simpler, saying, 'Yes, they have a dad, their dad lives in their house,' and she nods, satisfied. 'Have you got a dad?' I ask. She shakes her head. 'Passed away.' 'That was sad,' I say. She nods.*

May explained that as an in-law she didn't really count. 'Lily was totally family orientated. She knew exactly who was in the family, and it was only blood relatives. If I asked her whether she would like to go for a drive, she would answer to Bob that a drive would be nice,' May remembered with a hearty laugh. Despite this apparent rejection May was utterly dedicated to Lily, taking her to all her own family events and visiting her faithfully three or four times a week in the hospice. She was an important and stable figure in Lily's life.

Lily lived at the residential care home for 15 years, but she never really regarded it as her home. Home was where her family lived. Her family and support workers said that she didn't really have any friends. Bob felt that she merely tolerated the other residents in her new home, and looked to the staff for support and friendship. It was her brother she really wanted. Whenever Bob left her after a visit at the hospice, she wanted to know exactly when he would be back. 'I am allowed to go, as long as I promise when I will next be back. And woe the day that I am five minutes late…' He laughed, then added, looking very serious, 'She was always worried that she would be abandoned, that she would be all alone.'

The importance of families

Dame Cicely Saunders, who founded the modern hospice movement, regularly pointed out the importance of families. 'Death should be a family affair,' she wrote. 'Spouse, children and loved ones are all involved... People need dignity in death, and the dignity is in belonging; to your family and to society' (Saunders 2006, pp.239–240). Michael Young and Lesley Cullen, who spent several years listening to 14 terminally ill people and their families in East London, noted:

> Friends mostly drifted away, paying visits at the start of the illness and tailing off thereafter... On the whole the main work was left to the family who had so much more of the past to share. However sadly, they were together following the course of the disease week by week. (Young and Cullen 1996, p.66)

Parents and siblings, not partners and children

There was a striking difference between the important family relationships of people with learning disabilities and those of people in the general population. The people in the Veronica Project were middle aged if not older: a time in life when many people in the general population have acquired partners and children. When people develop serious illness they are usually able to rely on these partners and children; in Young and Cullen's study, wives and daughters were particularly important in providing physical and emotional support. People without partners or children often build up a supportive network of one or more committed friends.

People with learning disabilities rarely benefit from such networks. It is still highly unusual for them to share their lives with a sexual partner.

The lack of partners and children meant that the most important family relationships consisted of parents and siblings. People's sense of belonging to their families was striking. This was clearly the case for Lily, who had lived with her family for most of her life and whose family had stayed in close contact; but it was also true for those who had not had contact with their families for many years. However close they might be to the paid carers who supported them in their daily lives, it was the families who had 'staying power'. Paid carers, however dedicated, did not stay around forever; people who lived in residential care settings had known a long succession of paid carers throughout their lives, with only a few keeping in touch after they left. Family, however, would always be there. It is where people belonged, where they shared history and could be confident of a shared future. For most families in the Veronica Project their relative with learning disabilities was very important. Even relatives who could not spend much time with the person had a strong emotional bond with him or her.

Siblings were particularly prominent in the Veronica Project, which was probably a reflection of people's age. After their parents died and they realised that the person had no one else, brothers and sisters assumed a crucial role, sometimes with a sense of inevitability. The cancer diagnosis prompted many siblings to be even more involved; they acted as a support system and advocate.

In-laws became part of the family, too. In the stories of both Lily Lamb and Vincent Sweeney, the sister-in-law takes a central place. The spouses of siblings had become as safe as the siblings themselves: they would not move out of the person's life. One of the most committed family carers in this study was Joy, who had married Sally Burnett's father when Sally was a young teenager.

Vincent put into words what it was about the family that was so important. A year after we first met, he apologised for always talking about his brother and sister-in-law.

> *'It just shows how important they are,' I tell him. 'You've gone through so much. With this cancer. And also with your whole life. It hasn't been easy, and they...' Vincent finishes the sentence for me: 'They have always been there for me.'*

Jane Hubert, who carried out research with men with severe learning disabilities who had spent most of their lives on a locked ward of a long-stay institution, was struck by the way these men – many of whom barely spoke – still saw themselves as someone's son or brother, and craved a link with their families (Hubert and Hollins 2006). I found a similar need among people who had lived their lives in institutions. Whenever I visited Nick Ballard, the people he lived with surrounded me, tugging at my sleeve, desperately trying to communicate some important messages. After I first visited this home, I wrote about Nick's fellow residents:

She doesn't speak, but uses heavily repeated signs. I understand her signs for 'brother' and 'sister', but to be absolutely sure she finally writes her brother's full name and surname (and later, her own) on a piece of paper and shows it to me. She follows this information by writing 'Dad died'... But the most desperate attempts at telling me facts about her life come from another woman, seemingly in her sixties. She doesn't speak either, except in very crude noises, relying heavily on signs. I can occasionally work out what the sounds mean. She is desperate to tell me about her family too. She mimes a wedding ring, children, sitting on a knee; she points out the window, shouts 'Mummy', mimes crying, points towards heaven... I am not sure I completely understand, but what is clear is that she has, or had, a family, and that this is of crucial importance to her.

Families felt guilty

Family relationships were often complex. The birth of a child with disabilities has a profound effect on the relationships between parents and siblings. Parents could be deeply attached and protective of their needy and vulnerable child, and their sense of care and protectiveness never left them. People urged Mrs Davies to 'cut the apron strings' and be less protective of John, but she never did. The boy who, in her own words, 'always stayed close' was intrinsically linked to her sense of self; quite literally, she couldn't live without him.

People who had spent their childhood with a sibling with learning disabilities remembered, on the one hand, a simple acceptance of their 'different' brother or sister; and on the other hand, resentment about the extra attention their parents gave this disabled child, the way their sibling 'got away with murder', the way they themselves were sometimes expected to look after the disabled child or make allowances for him or her. They recognised, though, that much of this was simply the stuff of normal sibling rivalry. Bob said:

> 'I think I was aware, somehow, that she was handicapped, but to be honest it was just the way it was. She was my sister. I suppose I didn't always like to put up with her, like sometimes, when my mum used to say, "Go and play with Lily for half an hour, I need to do the cooking," but I think that was just me not wanting to play with my little sister, I'd rather be off with my own friends.'

In their childhood relationships with their brothers and sisters, people with learning disabilities were possibly the most 'normal' they would ever be, the most accepted simply for who they were.

There were feelings of guilt for letting their family member be taken into care. Only one woman, Pauline Deweert, lived with her family at the time of the cancer diagnosis; others had moved into residential care settings and, if possible, into their own homes. Many relatives had, at some point in their lives, contemplated the possibility of letting the person with learning disabilities live with them. Even when they acknowledged that this had not been possible, maybe not even what the person wanted, they wondered about it when cancer struck. Should life's choices have been different?

There were also feelings of guilt about not being more involved in the person's life. As Dimas Ferreira lay in his hospital bed, dying, his elderly aunt commented on the ever-changing team of support workers. Mrs Lopez met Dimas for the first time 14 years ago, when she 'took over' the visits from Dimas' grandmother who had moved back to her native Portugal ('Someone had to do it'). She had since built a deeply caring relationship with him that was important and meaningful to both of them. She said: 'I sometimes wonder whether it is fair that nobody stayed around for him. I should have visited him more. But I have a busy life. I do think I should have seen him more often.'

Feelings of guilt and regret were most painful where people had moved into institutional care in early childhood. Brothers and sisters recognised that their parents were not given a choice, that bringing up a child with learning disabilities at home was a difficult choice to make in those days, one that was frowned upon and advised against by the medical world. There was little support for parents of disabled children.

Marion Prentice was sent to live in an institution when she was diagnosed with Down's syndrome at the age of six months. Her sister Sarah, who was born the following year, only learnt of Marion's existence when she was in her late teens. She worked hard at building a relationship. Whenever she could she tried to make the ten-hour round trip to where Marion lived, to support Marion at her hospital appointments. She reflected with sadness on the lost years.

> 'I've always wanted a sister. Always. I longed for a sister when I was younger. And now I've got one. I've got a lovely sister, and I find it almost too painful to think about the life that could have been... When I was pregnant, I did think, if my child had Down's syndrome, I would just have her. And I did think about what that would do to my mother. If I knew I was going to have a child with Down's syndrome, would that be a criticism of her? I couldn't talk about that with her. Years later I did mention it to my mum, and she said, "Don't be silly, of course I wouldn't have minded. I would have loved a baby with Down's."'

This reflection is significant. It demonstrates the painful decisions families have to make about the care of their children with learning disabilities, but it also shows that a lack of visiting does not necessarily indicate a lack of love or care. When Marion's mother visited her daughter in the institution, she was told by the staff, 'You have to say to yourself that Marion is dead.' It is not difficult to see how contact between family members is thus lost.

The family of Ben Edwards, who moved into a long-stay institution when he was in his early teens, also had limited contact with him for several decades. Contact was restored due to the encouragement of staff at the residential care home he had now moved into. Ben's brother explained:

> 'It sounds awful, but those large hospitals really weren't very nice places. Big wards, lino, all very medical, and then you had all kinds of disabilities there... My mother is 90 now. It is difficult at her age... She sees him sometimes, but I think she still doesn't want to become too attached.'

Memories of children sent to live in long-stay institutions can be deeply painful, and the return of adult sons and daughters to community settings – as happened for Dimas, Ben, Ursula, Nick and Marion – is not always a straightforward moment of joy for families. Can this person really cope in society? Will he be safe and well cared for? Will society accept him? Dimas Ferreira's aunt said, 'I worried how people would react to him.' There are also some profound and difficult implications when people move back into society, as Jane Hubert explains:

> Once a child, or adult, has been committed to a long-term institution, how can they, years later, be brought back into society without indicting the family...? Such a move must carry with it the uncomfortable and, perhaps for some, unbearable implication that this person was not, and thus had really never been, beyond the social pale... Their young children, when they entered the institution, died a social death... To bring them back into the social world is too painful to contemplate. No one really wants to resurrect their dead. (Hubert 2000, p.205)

Although most paid carers tried to involve families, there could be a sense of blame towards them, particularly if the person with learning disabilities had been institutionalised. One support worker said:

> 'He is very insecure. I think it's because he was just left there by his family. I don't blame them, but...well...yes, I *do* blame them. I don't blame them for putting him in there, because it was probably very difficult at home; but I do blame them for not visiting him.'

Apart from feelings of guilt, there were feelings of anger and distress at the unfairness of cancer. This was felt by relatives and paid carers alike. 'He has had such a hard life, and now he's got this. Cancer. It's not fair.' The illness brought out a strong desire to protect. Life was difficult enough for someone with learning disabilities; that person shouldn't have to cope with cancer as well.

Paid carers didn't always recognise the importance of families

To understand the impact of family relationships and their importance towards the end of life, it is vital to understand the place of someone with learning disabilities in his or her family. It took me a while to realise this. Only as I met more of the relatives, and listened to those people with learning disabilities who could speak, did I begin to appreciate the vital role of family relationships in the meaning of someone's life and death.

Pete Carpenter was my first study participant, and I didn't talk to his sister Daphne at the time; his support workers were wonderfully committed and seemed to provide him with everything he needed. However, two years after Pete's death, 'families' had emerged as a major theme in the Veronica Project and I went back to meet with

Daphne. It was only then that I was able to put Pete's death into the context of his life, and understand how important it was that Pete was someone's son, someone's brother. In addition, Daphne was able to paint a picture of Pete's childhood that explained some of the ways he coped with his dying: his non-complaining nature, his continued love of steam trains and cycling magazines. Pete and Daphne's story appears later in this chapter.

Paid carers often did not understand the importance of families. Sometimes, they didn't even know of their existence. Richard Horwood had a key worker at his day centre who had worked with him for over two decades. When I told her how lovely it had been to meet Richard's brother and sister, this key worker was surprised: 'I didn't know he had siblings!' I had met the siblings during a review meeting. They had travelled a long distance to attend it, and when Richard's sister saw how unwell he was, she sat down and cried. Not only did he have siblings: these siblings were among the most significant people in his life. They didn't see each other often, but they were devastated by his illness.

Who 'owns' the person?

Relationships between families and paid carers were not always easy. Support workers who looked after someone with learning disabilities day after day usually got to know that person intimately. Their deep understanding of the person's character – people's likes and dislikes, the way they communicated – sometimes led them to believe that the person 'belonged' to them. 'We are his family now,' many support workers said.

Indeed, the close bonds many such carers formed with the people they supported were hugely important. Several relatives expressed their appreciation of this, particularly of staff who had stayed around for many years. But relatives could also see that paid carers were not committed for life. However closely involved, as Dimas' aunt had said, they didn't stay around forever. *Both* paid carers and families had an important part to play in people's lives, and these parts were not mutually exclusive. Tensions arose when carers assumed that they had 'rights' over someone that others didn't have, courtesy of their intense caring role, or of their blood relationship.

Lily's brother Bob was always careful not to criticise Lily's carers, whatever he thought of them privately. He sometimes had to bite his tongue. 'I try to work with them,' he said, realising that this was the best way to ensure good care for Lily. It worked: Lily's carers respected him and always involved him.

In some cases, there was a clear mutual respect between families and paid carers, with each side appreciating the importance of the other in the person's life. This was evident at the funeral of Ben Edwards where Ben's brother gave a heartfelt tribute to the staff at Ben's home:

> 'His was a very large family – one much wider than the one he was born into. It was one which grew and grew with those he lived with and all those who nurtured and cared for him…
>
> You took him out to the shops, the cinema, the circus, the fair, open air concerts, pubs and restaurants. You took him on summer holidays, swimming, on boat trips and even flying in light aircraft. You took photographs and made albums for him – and now us – to remember those happy times. You threw parties at Christmas and birthdays…
>
> And when he became ill, you took him to endless hospital appointments and stayed with him through the night in Accident and Emergency. You reassured him when he had to endure sometimes painful and frightening treatment and made sure he did not feel alone in the hospital wards. And you mashed his food and tended him through the night, so that he never had to part from his home.
>
> You cared for him as one of your own family. You always made my mother, sisters, brothers and I welcome at Ben's home, and we have a huge debt of gratitude for all you have done for us and thank you from the bottom of our hearts for enriching Ben's life with your unceasing care and devotion. Without doubt the past 15 years have been some of the happiest of his life.'

These words from Ben's brother were matched by a tribute from one of his support workers, recognising the importance of family:

> 'His family meant the world to him and he spoke of them often with great pleasure and pride. He loved them so dearly… I hope it gives some comfort to know how very much we cared

> for Ben and how he found happiness and true friendship in his other home.'

This was in sharp contrast to the feelings of Jason, the manager of Dimas Ferreira's home. Jason was Dimas' closest carer. He had known Dimas for the past five years. Jason was furious when Dimas' father came to the funeral. The father had moved to Thailand decades ago. Jason said afterwards:

> 'His father had no right to be there. He hasn't been to visit Dimas since he was 12 years old. Why did he suddenly come to the funeral? He should have come earlier. And he didn't stay, he just went straight back to Thailand that evening. It wasn't appropriate for all these family members to do readings and things when they never even bothered to come and see Dimas. Only his sister and his great-aunt should have been there, they were the only ones who kept in touch.'

However, I do not know, and neither could the care staff, how Dimas' estranged family felt about him. Maybe, like Marion's mother who didn't visit her but kept longing for a baby with Down's syndrome, Dimas' father had never stopped thinking about him. And maybe it hadn't occurred to Jason that of all the people at Dimas' funeral, only his non-visiting relatives had known him for longer than 14 years. Dimas' father was the only person who could have remembered Dimas as a small child.

The story of Pete Carpenter exemplifies all the issues discussed so far, and illustrates the importance of listening to families.

Pete Carpenter and his sister Daphne

Pete was 66 years old. Although his speech was limited to single words and short sentences, his severe learning disabilities were not immediately obvious. He had a gift for body language, copying conversational styles and gestures, mumbling along. His mimicking of other people's body language was so convincing that strangers often didn't realise the limitations of his speech and comprehension.

Pete enjoyed everything to do with English working-class life. He loved seeing dustbin men, builders, road menders and train drivers. He cheered at miners on television. He was a man of many enthusiasms. Skips, roll-up cigarettes and working men's cafés. Bikes, trams and trains. He listened to jazz, Acker Bilk and Lonnie Donegan, getting out his spoons to tap along. Pete taught generations of foreign support workers the essence of British Life, supervising the cooking of bacon and eggs for breakfast ('Bacon 'n' eggs, boys!'). He would explain in detail the workings of steam trains, leaving the poor staff desperately flicking through their dictionaries. He had smoked roll-ups since he was a child and wanted to be 'one of the boys'. His support workers controlled the amount he smoked; if left to his own devices, they said, he would smoke them so fast that he would literally make himself sick. In his younger years, it was his mother who held the cigarette papers.

But most of all, Pete loved work. One of his set phrases, frequently repeated, was 'Work in the morning, work, boys, work, work, work in the morning!' His support workers joked that much of his own work was done by osmosis, watching others work, standing around with tea and a cigarette, commenting on how well 'we' were doing. His eyes would light up and he would start chatting whenever he saw a worker in the street, particularly men in dirty overalls and hard hats. If he decided he wanted someone for a friend, he gave him or her no choice. He would be happy and cheerful every time he saw that person, and simply take no notice if he or she ignored him or responded negatively. This was how he made so many friends in the street: he greeted workmen and shopkeepers cheerfully every single day, as if they were the very person he had been longing to meet. Inevitably, these people would eventually relent and start chatting to him when they saw him. The man in the street he admired most was the owner of the bicycle shop, or 'the Bike Man' as Pete called him. At Pete's fiftieth birthday party, a group of support workers formed a jazz band, calling themselves 'The Bacon 'n' Egg Boys'; the Bike Man and his son turned up with a gift of a brand new bicycle.

For the past 25 years Pete had lived in a staffed residential care home where he made many friends. Support workers stayed in touch with him years or even decades after they left, and many travelled to London for his funeral. He was an easy man to like, but there was also a deeper, darker side to him. At times, he became angry and distressed, sometimes blackening his face with soot and biting his finger. His difficulty in coping with the deaths of people around him stemmed, his support workers knew, from the pain of living with the deaths of his father and mother. It was the reason why David, a terminally ill fellow resident, was taken to a hospice to die. Pete could not possibly cope with a death in his own home. Pete's support workers realised that he had known a lot of pain in his life, both physically and emotionally, although only a few long-term staff members knew the details of his life story.

Pete was diagnosed with lung cancer with only a few months to live. His health and strength gradually slipped away. He surprised those around him with his apparent acceptance, never complaining, spending more and more time asleep. He wanted to keep going to his day centre ('Work in the morning, boys'), and his support workers took him, letting him sit and doze in his chair whilst others were busy around him. He enjoyed visits of old friends who came to sing his favourite songs in his room. Pete died at home, with his support workers around him.

Pete had grown up with his family. He had a sister, Daphne, and a brother-in-law, Dennis, who visited him a couple of times a year. Daphne came to see him just once during his final illness. Pete's carers asked her to visit more, but she found it unbearably difficult to see his decline and preferred to remember him the way he was. She was deeply distressed at Pete's funeral, and chose not to come to the interment of his ashes at the local cemetery. I had met Daphne briefly at a review meeting soon after Pete's cancer diagnosis, but two years after his death I contacted her again. 'I'm not sure she'll want to talk to you,' Pete's support worker predicted. 'It always took us ages to get hold of her. She didn't really want to know.' But Daphne was more than happy to meet me, warning me beforehand: 'I am always thinking about Pete. My husband and I talk about his home a lot, too. I have his picture on my wall... I tend to run away from memories, I think you will reduce me to tears.'

'What really upset me,' she began as I was settled on the sofa of her comfortable home, 'was that he was the way he was because of delayed delivery. He was a special brother, but...well, he was my only brother. I don't have anyone else. People don't understand that. I know I've got my children, but...' She trailed off, unable to explain in words the deep bond with someone who had shared her childhood.

Daphne was a year younger than Pete. There were two much older half-siblings, a brother and sister, children of their mother's first marriage whose father had died. The brother didn't keep in touch with Pete, and Daphne resented him for it. 'He would just send me a cheque at Christmas, saying, "Get Pete something from me." But my sister's husband Dennis got on really well with Pete. They were just like two boys, going camping together, playing about, falling over... It was lovely.' Pete's support workers had told me about Dennis, who kept in faithful contact with Pete over the years.

'When we were children,' Daphne continued, 'I didn't understand. I knew he was different but I didn't understand why. My parents never told me, and I think that was wrong. Pete got away with murder, and I didn't. I didn't think that was fair. If something was broken... "Who did that? Pete? Oh well, never mind. Daphne? You make sure you never do it again!" They made allowances for Pete, but not for me. I had quite a temper as a child, and I was furious. Pete used to cycle to the railway sidings. And it was *my* bike! I got it for my birthday, and then he took it and used it. My sister said, "Let him use it," but I didn't think it was fair. It was mine. But I had to let him use it... I can understand it now, but I didn't then. And in a funny way, these things never leave you. Sometimes I still feel like that. That things are not fair.

He was in hospital a lot when he was little. He had this problem with his feet, they pointed sideways. He had this contraption that had to be tightened at night. It was always hurting him. He was in so much pain. He shared a bedroom with his brother, and sometimes his brother couldn't bear listening to him in pain. He would tell Pete to stop it. Sometimes my mother would come in and loosen them.

My mother adored Pete, and did everything for him. Well, they both did, but I don't think my father could ever accept the way he was. Pete was an embarrassment to him. At first a disappointment, I think, and then an embarrassment. He wanted to hide Pete away. We used to go on camping holidays, staying in a caravan, and I'm not saying that was because of Pete's mental handicap, but it did limit us. And when Pete sat next to him in public, he would say [miming a stern voice and an elbow thump] "Be quiet! Behave yourself!" I think my father was a very private man. He didn't show his emotions. He never complained. When you say Pete was like that when he was ill, I am thinking, maybe he took after his father.

Pete didn't really have any friends of his own, but he would just be part of us. There was no traffic at the time, so we would all play out in the streets. Or he would cycle up to the station. It was the end of the line in those days, so the steam trains would arrive and they would load and unload the engines, and Pete would just spend all day there, watching. They all knew him.

He would often sit in his room, listening to his radio and his music. He just did his own thing. He always lived at home. Then my father died of cancer. He died at home. Pete was about 30 years old, and I think it was a terrifying experience for him. I don't think it was a good death, with a lot of pain. Pete never talked about it, but he knew Dad died of cancer.

After that it was just him and my mum. I visited quite a lot though, to help my mum out. I often thought, if something happens to Mum, what will happen to Pete? It will have to be me. I spoke about it to a social worker at the time, and she said, "We'll cross that bridge when we get there." But I always thought I'd never get married and have children. I thought I couldn't. I would have to look after Pete.

Then my mum died suddenly. It was horrible. Pete was on holiday at the time. They wouldn't let him see her. He was just dragged away. He went to a temporary home first, somewhere miles away. There were these awful social workers who said that they were doing the best for Pete. And they hadn't even met him! They said they knew all about him from his files. But how could that be the best for Pete, moving so far away, when all his friends were here? Of course there were all these things going around the family, "Maybe we should take him in," that sort of thing. I thought I would have him live with me, but I wasn't allowed. Social services wouldn't let me. They said I couldn't look after him properly, I was working and he needed 24-hour care. I don't think he did, really. We often left him to get on with things, and he would just go to his room and do his own thing. Or would I have left him alone in the house? I don't know... Maybe I would have given up work... But in the end, I am glad he went to that home. It was good for him. He made lots of friends there, and he came into his own, beginning to explore the world... I think if he had stayed with me, I would just have mollycoddled him. But I still feel guilty about it now.'

Pete came to see Daphne and her family a couple of times a year, and she visited him, too. However, she never found those visits easy. She didn't know how to cope with one of Pete's fellow residents, who had a habit of coming up close to everyone, including strangers, and kissing them. With hindsight, Daphne felt she should have asked the support workers for help in dealing with this; but her way of coping was simply by not visiting very often.

Two years after his death, Pete was never far from her thoughts. 'I was really, really angry at his funeral,' she said, and then asked herself aloud: 'Why was I angry? Who was I angry with? I suppose I was angry with Pete. Yes, I was. I was furious. I remember at the end of the funeral, in the end in the crematorium, everyone took a handful of wood shavings to put on his coffin. I can't quite remember what I did with it but I think I threw it at the coffin. "How *dare* you die," I thought. "How dare you! Leave me like that!" And I still think that now. I have his photograph on the dressing table in my bedroom, and every evening I look at him, and I still get a lurch in my stomach. I still feel angry. "Why did you die?" I think. "Why did you leave me? Where are you now?" I feel guilty, too. It's a terrible guilt, even now, and maybe it will never go away. I know I shouldn't feel guilty but I can't help it.'

Later, when I saw Pete's support worker again, I told her how Daphne was still missing Pete. The support worker was incredulous. 'Is she? But it's been two years! And she only saw him twice a year!'

Friends

Lack of friends

Friends can be an important source of support during times of hardship. Many people with learning disabilities have difficulty making and sustaining friendships, because they often depend on their families and care staff to meet or stay in contact with other people. Those who were able to make phone calls had a clear advantage here. For Vincent Sweeney, the telephone was a life line. Lack of funds could be a problem. One day, John Davies felt very low, because the credit on his telephone had run out and he couldn't talk to his friends.

Most people, though, had very few friends, if any. Some had moved away from peers again and again, with little influence over where they lived or who they saw; some had lived isolated lives with their families; some lacked confidence and self-esteem, the roots of which lay in their childhoods when they were bullied at school. Now in her fifties, Pauline Deweert said:

> 'I don't have any friends. I did have a friend at school. But she wasn't very nice. She had sticking out teeth, and people always called her names. She wasn't nice to people. She used to stick her tongue out at people all the time. I don't see her now.'

Some people with learning disabilities did have friends, but they depended on others to arrange visits, particularly when they were ill. Their friends with learning disabilities usually couldn't visit without the help of a carer. People had little power over such visiting arrangements.

Bob and May asked Lily's support workers not to bring Lily's fellow residents into the hospice during her final weeks: they wanted them to remember Lily 'as she was'.

Sally Burnett was distressed that so few of her friends with learning disabilities visited her at the hospice. I only learnt of the extent of her friendships at her funeral, which was attended by a very large crowd of people with and without learning disabilities, who spoke of her fondly. Sally's friend from the athletics club took a long time to tell me, 'I wish...Sally...was still...alive.'

Hundreds of people attended Vincent Sweeney's funeral, but when he was ill he was very lonely; his friends didn't visit him when he could no longer go out as much as he used to.

Support workers were seen as friends

People who lived in residential care services often considered the staff who supported them to be their friends. As was the case with Lily Lamb, most of these residents focused their attention on the staff, not on the other people with learning disabilities. Some people in the Veronica Project had known the people they lived with for decades; both Ben Edwards and Nick Ballard, for example, had moved into their residential care home together with some others they had grown up with in institutions. However, if they had developed close relationships with their fellow residents, this was not obvious to me as an outsider, or to the staff whom I asked about it. Nick Ballard seemed to see them as competitors, people who took staff's attention away from him; other people with learning disabilities were often afraid of him.

The relationships with staff members were mostly warm and caring. However, the relationship between a support worker and someone with learning disabilities is rarely an equal relationship between two adults. Mary illustrated this very clearly when she described her deep feelings of love for Nick Ballard: 'He is like my pet.'

The support worker usually dictates the terms of the relationship, including the level of intimacy. One key element of friendship is *reciprocity*, where both friends have a need of each other. It is this lack of reciprocity that makes relationships between staff and people with learning disabilities different from most friendships. The support worker may have a need of the person with learning disabilities for a variety of reasons: the need to give love and care, the need to enjoy the person's affections, the need to be enriched by the person's life – but these reasons do not usually include a personal need for friendship. People with learning disabilities have fewer opportunities than most of us to be a giving and supportive partner in a reciprocal friendship.

People with learning disabilities whose friendships consist mostly of staff are vulnerable to loss. Support workers leave. They may stay in touch, but lifelong friendships are rare. Vincent Sweeney experienced this, a continuous disappointment because the people he considered as important as friends moved away, or dropped him from their caseload: his social worker, his hospice nurse, his learning disability nurse.

Friendship under scrutiny

Vincent Sweeney made friends with Frank, a fellow patient at the hospice day centre. It was an intense friendship. Frank and Vincent were two lonely men, both living alone, both frightened, both unable to sleep at night. They started ringing each other throughout the long and lonely nights, every hour, on the hour. Once, Frank rang three times during the hour I spent at Vincent's flat. The nurses at the hospice were concerned; they disapproved of the friendship. 'Frank is talking about Vincent as if he is his boyfriend, but I don't think Vincent sees it like that.' They worried that it might be abusive. I once asked Vincent outright whether Frank was his boyfriend, and he was taken aback: 'No! No, I'm not gay. He is just a really good friend.' However, I felt uncomfortable even about my need to ask. Was it actually anyone's business to judge people's friendships? Vincent was clear why he valued Frank's friendship so much: 'He is like me. He is lonely. Sometimes he rings me up too early, and it wakes me up, but it doesn't matter.'

When Frank died, Vincent was devastated.

> 'I don't think I will ever get over it. I've lost a part of my life... I miss him, you know. I miss the time we spent together. We would go to the cinema for a couple of hours, then I would come home in the evening and we would spend three hours on the phone... It's all gone.'

What was striking about Vincent's friendship with Frank was that Frank needed Vincent as much as Vincent needed Frank. This opportunity to fulfil the need for a reciprocal relationship with someone who is not a member of your family was very rare among the men and women in the Veronica Project. Concerns about abuse or exploitation may well have prevented some people with learning disabilities from developing independent friendships, thus robbing them of the chance of a friend's support at the end of life.

Because sick and disabled people have to depend on others, many aspects of their lives, including their friendships, are subject to close scrutiny.

Fellow residents

Fellow residents were usually kept out of the way; few were given the opportunity to help look after the dying person that they had known for so long. Karen, Lily Lamb's home manager, was amazed at my suggestion that the other residents could maybe help by bringing Lily her drink: 'That's a wonderful idea! I never thought of that. Yes, I think Laksha would really enjoy that.' It seemed that here, as in friendships in general, people with learning disabilities lacked opportunities to give rather than to receive. They were dependent on others.

Residential care staff were concerned about the effect of the illness and dying on people's fellow residents. The support workers usually told them simply that the person was 'not well'; sometimes they also mentioned 'cancer'. Support workers wondered whether they should explain more, but few fellow residents asked any further questions.

Staff sometimes felt guilty about the extra time they had to spend with the ill person, but other residents mostly seemed to accept that their house mate needed more help, and that the staff had less time for them.

Some carers noticed clear reactions in the residents. After Ben Edwards died, Yanna, his home manager, said of a fellow resident with severe learning disabilities: 'The home is empty without Ben. I think they all feel it. Jamie keeps going into Ben's room, just standing in his room, looking around.'

Maureen, who had moderate learning disabilities, also showed feelings of concern. She lived with Pete Carpenter and had known him for 25 years. The support workers had been open about Pete's cancer, and had told his house mates that he wouldn't get better. Maureen did not usually mince her words. She grabbed my hand on my first visit: 'I thought it was me you come to see! I don't need seeing to. It's Pete that needs seeing to. I told him, I told him not to smoke, but he wouldn't listen!'

Towards the end of Pete's life, he was no longer able to manage the stairs and spent a few nights sleeping in the sitting room. A long-term, trusted member of staff at Maureen's day centre told the support workers that Maureen had expressed fear and distress about this. Maureen was frightened that she would be in the room when Pete died. She had said: 'It's all right for you, you go home to your own house at the end of the day. I have to sit there and watch it.'

The home manager was shocked to hear this: he wasn't aware of the extent of Maureen's distress. 'She is really generous with Pete,' he said. 'She never complains, and never moans at him.'

In other homes, carers doubted that people were much missed by their peers when they died. When Nick was ill, Mary said: 'They sometimes ask: "Where's Nick?" And we say, "He is not well, he is in hospital." And they seem to be OK with that, they just forget.' After Nick's and Ursula's deaths, she reflected:

> 'They seemed fine. They had no reaction at all. They just seemed to accept it. They never asked any questions. They just carried on as normal... We do talk about Ursula and Nick sometimes, just in conversation. Their pictures are still up on

> the wall, and when visitors ask, the others just say, "That's Ursula, she is gone now, she's dead."'

Dimas Ferreira lived with people with severe and profound learning disabilities, none of whom could speak. His carers doubted whether any of them would actually miss Dimas, or even notice that he was gone.

I wondered about this. The ability of people with learning disabilities to grieve is not dependent on their cognitive ability (Oswin 1991), and it would seem strange that people who have lived together for decades would not miss each other. It is also possible that some people with learning disabilities were sensitive to the huge support needs of the ill person and to the stress and distress of their support workers; maybe they wanted to protect them by not making any demands themselves. This was illustrated clearly by Veronica Donaghey, the woman who inspired the Veronica Project and whose cancer story was made into a book. When she told her story, she remembered a good friend who had died.

> The day of the funeral I had to be strong for Paula, Vera [friends] and Catherine [community nurse]... It was a burial. I don't think Paula and Vera had gone to one where the coffin goes down in the ground. I had to be strong for them as well. I couldn't cry then. I sometimes cry now. (Donaghey et al. 2002, p.50)

Summary

Families

- The families of people with learning disabilities were of crucial importance in their lives. This was true even for those who had limited contact with their relatives. Social care staff, however committed, came and went; family was there forever, creating a mutual sense of belonging.
- In the absence of partners and children, relationships with parents, brothers and sisters were extremely important. Many siblings were strongly committed to this relationship. In-laws were part of this important family network, too.

- Many families felt guilty about not having been more present in their relative's life, and about their relative having been taken into care. Such feelings of guilt were heightened during the terminal illness and after death.
- Paid carers (support workers) did not always recognise the important place of families. There could be tensions about who 'owned' the person with learning disabilities; some support workers felt that they themselves had become 'family', and therefore had more rights over the person.

Friends

- Most people with learning disabilities had very few friends.
- People with learning disabilities are often dependent on others to help them maintain friendships. Most people with learning disabilities lost contact with friends when they were ill; sometimes, friends (especially friends with learning disabilities) were unable to visit, or discouraged from visiting.
- Those living in residential care services often saw the support workers as their friends, and related mostly to them (rather than to other people with learning disabilities). However, people with learning disabilities lacked power in their relationships with staff. These were not mutual, reciprocal friendships. The need of people with learning disabilities to have their support workers as their friends makes them vulnerable to loss when the support worker leaves.
- Some people who made friends independently met with disapproval from carers of their friendships.
- Some support workers did not think that people's fellow residents were much affected by the person's illness and death. Most fellow residents did not make their feelings clear, although a few were distressed and frightened.

CHAPTER 5

Unprepared Services, Inexperienced Carers

For most of the staff in learning disability services, working with someone who had cancer was a new experience. They had never been with anyone who was dying before, and supporting someone with end-stage cancer was difficult for them. Conversely, for the health care professionals, doctors and nurses in hospitals, hospices and nursing homes, working with someone who had learning disabilities was unfamiliar.

This chapter puts the spotlight on paid carers, illustrating their struggles and triumphs. The main focus is on residential care services. Seven people lived in residential care homes where they were supported by paid carers 24 hours a day. There were examples of very good practice, as well as times when things did not go well. It is worth looking at the carers' experiences in some detail, as they illustrate the challenges faced by residential care services.

First of all, here is what happened in the homes of Lily Lamb and Pete Carpenter.

Lily Lamb and her carers

Lily's parents started making provision for her future by putting her name down for a residential home. It was the 1970s; long-stay hospitals for people with learning disabilities were closing, and a number of new community homes were being opened in the local area. One of the homes accepted her, but when Lily's mother died suddenly of a heart attack, plans for the move were shelved for a decade. She finally moved into the residential home when her father became too old and frail to support her. There were six other residents at the home.

The home was part of a larger organisation of residential care homes, with overall management support. When Lily's cancer was diagnosed the team of carers included Karen, the manager who had worked at the home for five years and had recently been promoted after the previous manager left; and William, who had worked at the home since Lily arrived there 15 years earlier. Four experienced members of staff had left in the few months before Lily's diagnosis, and the home relied on agency staff. Only Karen and William knew Lily well. There were usually two support workers present during the day, but only one support worker was on duty in the evening and during the night. Now that Lily's care needs had become more complex, Karen tried to make sure that either she herself or William was on duty at any given time, as no one else knew Lily well enough. My notes describe my first visit to the home.

> *I express my amazement and concern. Isn't this a lot to take on? What happens when they have days off, holidays, or are off sick? I suggest that caring for Lily must be stressful, because it is a journey into the unknown for them, and they also have to support the other residents. Both immediately agree. They discuss together how they cannot see when they can take time off; at the same time, Karen says that they must take their days off. They cannot keep going for months without a break. When I look rather concerned to hear that there is only one staff member in the evenings, Karen seems to realise: 'Actually I don't know how I'm going to manage at the weekend, I don't think we can do it...' When Lily needs the commode, for example, staff can manage it on their own, but 'You can't rush her.' My mind boggles. How on earth do they manage to give adequate support to seven residents in these conditions?*

The district nurses agreed to come in and help Lily to have a wash in the mornings, and a palliative care nurse visited for advice on pain control. It was the uncertainty about how to manage Lily's pain that caused the support workers the most stress, and they were desperate for advice and support. Were they doing the right thing? When should they be thinking about giving extra painkillers? Lily had started taking morphine tablets, but the staff didn't know what to do when the pain was still bad. There was no top-up morphine in the house. They tried to telephone the palliative care nurse but could not get hold of her. My notes continue:

> *There are other pressures. A sink caused a flood last night. The day centre rings to say that the rest of the residents are on their way back home because of a power cut. Karen puts her head in her hands: 'Oh no! Oh no, we needed to...' 'We're supposed to have supervision this afternoon,' William reminds her. 'Oh well,' says Karen, 'let him see what it is really like. He hasn't been very much help, he's only rung once to see how things are going.' He, apparently, is the line manager.*

A week later, however, things were considerably easier. As the extent of Lily's needs became obvious, support was put in place.

> *Karen is looking and feeling much more relaxed, and readily admits this. The change is mainly due to a sharp increase in the support they are getting. District nurses come twice a day. Marie Curie night sitters have been arranged, and have just started doing a 'waking night' with her each night – although it emerges that last night, they rang at 10pm to say they couldn't make it due to family problems, so the staff member on duty ended up being awake for most of the night. Karen sends her home as soon as she realises this: 'You must be knackered.'*
>
> *The hospice has organised all these services, and Karen is delighted. Her own manager is also realising how things stand. When I told Karen that I had been wondering how she'd managed at the weekend, as the only member of staff after 7pm, she smiled: 'I got extra staff.'*

But it was never easy. A hospital bed arrived, but there was no space for a hoist or even a wheelchair in Lily's tiny bedroom. Lily was clearly distressed and kept saying that she should be in hospital. It seemed that she was confused about the fact that she was at home when she was clearly not well. In the end, her continuing pain problems prompted a transfer to the hospice. 'The nurses couldn't manage the care any more,' Karen said. 'The pain was so bad, they just couldn't do anything with her.'

Lily had been at home from hospital for three weeks, and would be in the hospice for a further eight weeks before she died. Senior managers of her residential home made it clear that she could not return. The carers felt that they could no longer support her. Lily's family reluctantly agreed that the home was no longer suitable, but they were distressed by the swiftness with which the organisation that had promised her a home for life 'washed their hands of her', as May, her sister-in-law, described it. They lamented the fact that the carers were no longer allowed to visit Lily in work time. The care agency did not have enough flexibility in their staffing levels to enable such visits. Karen and William did visit, but only in their free time.

The fact that Lily's condition became reasonably stable was an issue of some concern. The hospice was not a long-stay facility, and Lily's prognosis was uncertain. She could deteriorate at any time, but she could also live for a good number of months. The question of where she should be cared for, once her pain was controlled, began to trouble people's minds. Lily herself was possibly the only person who was not aware of this question, or at least did not show any concerns about it.

The hospice encouraged Bob and May to start looking at nursing homes for Lily. This caused them a huge amount of worry. They visited a few nursing homes, accompanied by Karen who had offered to come with them on her day off; but they didn't find anywhere suitable. The hospice nurses quietly campaigned for Lily to stay at the hospice, where she felt safe. There was really nowhere else suitable for her to go.

Lily liked the hospice from the moment she arrived. She loved the large, bright single room, with the adjustable bed and plenty of space for a wheelchair and hoist, as well as two comfy armchairs for her visitors. There were usually at least two nurses available when she needed them, patiently helping her to sit up, lie down, move her legs, give her a drink. It was 'handy', she said. She wasn't sure how long she would stay in the hospice, or whether she would go back home again, but she was very clear what she herself preferred. 'Stay here.'

There was a guilty sense of relief when her condition deteriorated, because it meant that she could stay in the hospice. But Lily's family were galvanised into writing to the residential care organisation where Lily had lived for 15 years. Bob wrote:

> 'Despite the best efforts of the [learning disability care home] staff, they are not trained with the appropriate nursing skills.

Based on our experience the nursing homes lack the appropriate learning disability skills... Consequently the residents fall into a gap and are at risk of not receiving the necessary medical and psychological support when they most need it... I am eternally grateful to the hospice for their help, but we should not rely on the hospice to fill the gap. I do not wish to criticise, but I feel that there is a major concern here and a potential problem looming.'

Pete Carpenter and his carers

Pete Carpenter, whose life story was described in the previous chapter, also lived at a residential care home. Pete died at home. It was a gentle and peaceful death. Pete was lovingly supported, but it wasn't easy for the support workers, and I sometimes wondered whether the cost to them was too high.

Pete's home was an ordinary house in an ordinary street, shared with Maureen and Jenny who also had learning disabilities. They were supported by a team of five support workers, led and managed by Ramesh who had been there a couple of years. Maria had also worked at the home for several years; the other members of staff had joined the team in the past year. None was English. The home was part of a wider organisation of group homes within the same local area, with strong links of mutual support and friendship, and with overall management support.

When Pete was diagnosed with cancer and his carers were told that he only had a few months left to live, they tried to plan ahead. The senior management team called a meeting with all his support workers. The most difficult question the carers grappled with at this meeting was 'to tell or not to tell', but there was a list of other potential problems: how to cope with Pete's increasing weakness, his pain, weight loss and continued smoking – there was general agreement that smoking was OK now, though they had previously encouraged him to cut down. There was concern for the support workers: would they cope, emotionally, with supporting a dying man? The GP and the district nurses increased their input. The hospice nurse came to help with symptoms of pain and breathlessness, and to give the team advice and support. Yet despite all this planning and potential support, nobody was quite prepared for the rollercoaster of change that comes with end-stage cancer.

During the first weeks after his diagnosis, much of the carers' time was spent liaising with the hospital. They took Pete to several appointments, including a day-long stay for investigations. Decisions needed to be taken about whether these tests were necessary, and in Pete's best interest. Hospital doctors and the hospice nurse gave their opinion and advice about possible investigations, but it was left to the carers to decide. They found this difficult: they felt they needed to be good advocates for Pete, yet they lacked medical knowledge and confidence to ease their decision making.

In the meantime, Pete seemed content to be with his carers and friends, reminiscing together, listening to his favourite songs or sitting in companiable silence. He would regularly look up and catch their eye, smiling. However, when I returned after a three-week holiday his health had deteriorated significantly and he was much more tired. He still wanted to go to his day centre, but now stayed at home every morning, dozing. Pete was never told clearly that he was dying, and he didn't seem worried or upset about his rapidly declining health and abilities, although he sometimes panicked during an attack of breathlessness. The following extract from my field notes describes his condition a week before he died.

> *Pete is sitting in the conservatory. He looks much weaker than last week, with a poorer colour and noisy, laboured breathing. He looks up to acknowledge me, but doesn't smile; his face is slightly frowned. His upper body is heaving with the effort of breathing. However, when I ask him how he is, he says, 'All right.' And when I ask him whether he is feeling ill at all, he repeats 'I'm all right'...*
>
> *Pete takes out his cigarette box and tries to roll a cigarette. He can't do it. He keeps redistributing the tobacco, trying and failing to roll it, redistributing the tobacco again. He seems perfectly at peace with this age-old, familiar ritual, content just to sit there with the cigarette box on his lap and the paper in his hand. But after five minutes or so he holds his tobacco out to me: 'You do it.' He has never asked me this before, and I do it for him and light it.*
>
> *Pete asks for a couple of drinks. His tea has gone cold and I make him another one. He asks for orange juice, and I bring him that too. I leave him, and when I come back five minutes later he has the tea mug in his hand and has spilled the tea over his shoes. I clean it up.*

Pete does seem bothered by his frequent coughing, and in particular by the copious amounts of sputum he brings up, dribbling onto his clothes. The support workers are kind and gentle, telling him it doesn't matter and cleaning it up immediately.

Pete's upstairs bedroom was a problem. The team considered putting his bed downstairs, but dismissed this idea as being too disruptive for Maureen and Jenny, who would lose their sitting room. Putting in a stair lift would take too long. The difficulty with the stairs was never properly sorted out. When Pete did indeed become too weak to manage the stairs safely, he was still enjoying his visits to the café and to the day centre. The support workers were reluctant to confine him to his bedroom. There was also concern about his tendency to get up very early in the morning and totter down the stairs unsupervised. One night, a support worker found him asleep on the floor next to his bed. She was frightened by the change in his breathing, which stopped and started. She made him comfortable on the spot, using pillows and blankets. He then spent a couple of nights sleeping in the downstairs living room, in a hastily purchased armchair. The team decided that his bed should be brought downstairs after all, into the living room, as a temporary arrangement until he could no longer go out, at which point he could be nursed in his upstairs bedroom. This decision was supported by the senior management team, but it was not without difficulties. The manager who co-ordinated Pete's care had spoken to someone at social services, and had been told that there could be problems with allowing Pete to sleep in the living room. There were implications for the other residents, whose living space would be affected (and as I described earlier, Pete's house mate Maureen was indeed frightened to witness Pete's illness). As it happened – and this was considered lucky by many – Pete died at home a few days later, when both Maureen and Jenny were away for the weekend. His last couple of days were calm and peaceful, but it could have looked very different if he had lived another few weeks, or even another few days.

The support workers at Pete's home were deeply committed to him, giving him as much attention as they could, trying hard to ensure that he had the best possible care and that he could stay at home. Pete's illness was difficult and exhausting for them, both physically and emotionally. Ramesh frequently helped out on his day off, as did several other support workers. Kathleen, Pete's advocate and day centre manager, had been planning to leave her job, but now decided that she wanted to stay long enough to see Pete through his final illness. When I felt that Pete was entering his last weeks of life, I took Kathleen aside and talked to her about it.

Kathleen agrees, and cries on and off throughout our talk. She is obviously very much affected by Pete. She talks about waking up at 3.30am, thinking about Pete, unable to sleep. She is touched by him, and by the gentle way he is coping with his illness. She is upset by the fact that he went for the biopsy (she was on holiday at the time): 'I thought we had agreed that he wouldn't need to go through any more tests'... I am somewhat worried about her. Her own mother has died not very long ago. Kathleen has a deep emotional involvement, and very high standards and expectations. It is hard for her.

Only Kathleen happened to have any kind of medical training (she was a qualified nurse). All the other support workers struggled with their lack of knowledge and experience. This was most obvious in their dealings with pain. Pete was very good at hiding pain, and usually simply said 'I'm all right.' He would sometimes point at his chest and say 'Pain, pain', but it was difficult to get a consistent picture of how the pain affected him. Right from the start, Ramesh worried. How would they know Pete was in pain? Pete was initially given tablets to be used on an as-needed basis in addition to his regular painkillers, but how would Ramesh and his team know when it was OK to give them? Despite advice from the visiting hospice nurse, they all worried about giving too much or too little.

During his last weeks, even regular medication became difficult for Pete to take. The team was patient, but constantly worried about whether they would manage to help Pete take his medication, and whether it mattered if they couldn't.

When it is time for Pete's lunchtime medication, Ramesh (who is in fact on his day off) spends a calm, relaxed and gentle five minutes giving him morphine liquid in small bits on a teaspoon. Pete takes it willingly, but says, 'That's enough now' before it is finished. He keeps asking for a shave, so Ramesh suggests having a break from the medication. They go off into the bathroom together. It is only ten steps away, but Pete chooses to use his newly arrived wheelchair. When they come back, Pete gives him a full teaspoon of antibiotics, which Pete takes in licks and sips. This also takes several minutes; then he says firmly that he doesn't want any more now. There are still two teaspoons full of paracetamol left to take, but Ramesh doesn't give this.

Although the senior managers of the organisation expressed awareness early on that the team would need to be well supported, and offered the support workers regular opportunities to talk through their needs, there was no clear practical support in place for the rapid changes and emergencies of advanced cancer. After two months, the support workers were tired and frightened of what lay ahead, and Ramesh telephoned me. It was like an SOS: 'Irene, I think we need help.' He asked me to come and talk with him and the team about how they were managing. 'It would really help us. You have so much experience.' The hospice nurse had visited and talked through some of the team's worries, but she wasn't due to visit again until next week and didn't think it was necessary to come earlier.

When I sat down with the team, Ramesh admitted feeling particularly shaky about giving medication, which now sometimes took half an hour; but there were other issues, too.

There are questions about how Pete's condition will change, and ultimately, how Pete will die. A new support worker, who has only been here ten days, says anxiously how bad Pete's breathing was yesterday, and how Pete had looked quite panicked. The hospice nurse had advised giving tranquillisers on these occasions, making Ramesh worried about not knowing when to give it: when is Pete panicked enough? I tell them that Pete is not going to die of lack of breath in the middle of a panicked breathing attack. The support workers' response shows that this is in fact precisely what they had been worried about...they obviously had unrealistic images of how death happens, and were worried about Pete 'dying on them' unexpectedly.

The team relied on Maureen's night sitter to keep an eye on Pete too, but now Ramesh suddenly realised that the following day, this night sitter would not be here because Maureen was going on holiday. They did not otherwise have waking night staff. Ramesh tried to telephone his senior managers, but could not reach them. None of the emergency phones was switched on, and Ramesh said, exasperated, 'This is much more stressful than anything, trying to get hold of people. It really annoys me when they say I should take time and talk about my feelings, when what I really need is someone to answer the telephone when I need support for Pete.'

The senior management team and outside professionals acknowledged that the team needed a lot of support, practical as well as emotional, but did not act quickly enough when the support needs increased. I telephoned the hospice nurse, conscious of my tricky multiple roles as researcher and nurse with experience of palliative care. I told her that I had met with the team at their request. Her immediate reaction was annoyance: 'Why don't they talk to me? I told them they can ring me at any time, and I have already arranged to come in four days time.' I explained about the worries they had discussed with me. She seemed even more annoyed: 'That's a little bit naughty really. I went over all that with them… They keep asking me what to expect, and of course I can't tell them that, because nobody knows.' She thought the team was asking her about Pete's exact prognosis and manner of death, which was indeed impossible to predict; but it occurred to me that they actually needed to know what 'end of life' looked like and what the likely care needs were. This kind of information may be taken for granted by palliative care nurses, but support workers simply don't know about dying, and lie awake worrying about it.

Pete died quickly on a Sunday morning, two days after my meeting with the team. Ramesh telephoned me a couple of hours later, and in the evening I joined Pete's friends who had started gathering at his home. The support workers helped me to piece together what had happened.

It was the first time Pete didn't get out of bed. However, he was still lucid and talking, sitting up to take his medication before lunchtime. Although he looked much weaker, the support workers had no inkling that he was imminently dying. His breathing was clearly worse: it sounded more laboured, noisier, with more gaps. When Pete indicated between his legs, Ramesh understood that he had wet himself for the first time. Ramesh telephoned the hospice, but the nurse was out and would ring back later. Ramesh couldn't get hold of his senior managers. He began to worry to the point of panic. Pete was suddenly looking much worse. If this is how he is now, Ramesh thought, needing nursing care, then we really can't manage it. There was no support, no nurses available to come in, and a team not knowing what to do for the best.

Concerned about Pete's very rapid decline, Ramesh rang for an ambulance. 'It was funny really,' he told me later that day, with tears in his eyes and still shaking slightly. 'I kept saying, "Hello", it was like: "Hello?" "Hello!" "Hello?" – I couldn't get my words out clearly, like telling them that there was a fire or an accident.' In the meantime, the new support worker was sitting with Pete when he simply stopped breathing. Maria came in almost immediately and was the first to note that Pete had actually died.

The three support workers sat with Pete's body for 30 minutes before the ambulance arrived. The ambulance crew tried to resuscitate Pete (as they must, when called in to someone who shows no signs of life) and his body was then taken to hospital. Ramesh felt incredibly guilty and stupid for having telephoned the ambulance. In tears, he said, 'They did all those things, resuscitation, it wasn't nice. I feel really awful about it. But I've never seen someone die. I didn't know what it looks like. I feel really…' He was lost for words, indicating shakiness. 'I didn't know what was happening. I didn't know what to do. I panicked.'

Although Pete's death was as comfortable as it could have been, in familiar surroundings with staff who loved him, I felt frustrated that the team were left to cope on their own when so much support was potentially in place. There had been referrals to the hospice, Marie Curie nurses and district nurses. But of course deaths often cannot be planned, and Pete died much more quickly than anyone had anticipated. We had envisaged a period of reduced consciousness and dying, during which time procedures and extra support could be nicely planned. I realised how crucially important it is that teams are prepared for what lies ahead. They need to know what to expect at a death. They need to know what it looks like, what it might feel like, what they should do, and what they don't have to do. I thought the organisation had planned this, but they obviously failed to take on board what happens at the actual time of death, and they failed to plan what they wanted to do about the body.

The toll taken on the team became obvious in the months following Pete's death. Ramesh was physically exhausted and collapsed emotionally. He ended up taking a couple of weeks sick leave. He remained upset, feeling guilty and angry with himself for the episode with the ambulance. Ramesh was surprised at the impact Pete's illness had on him. He and the rest of his team found it hard to get used to the changes in the house, changed dynamics, changed routines. 'We keep expecting Pete to come downstairs mid-morning, but then remember that he is not here and we don't have to do anything.' Ramesh had some upheavals in his personal life as well, and decided to leave his job as home manager a few months after Pete died. He returned to become a member of the senior management team a year later. Two years after Pete's illness and death he looked back on it as a good experience, but an emotional one, that still brought tears to his eyes.

Other support workers struggled, too. One support worker became ill as soon as she had a holiday. She then had to return to her home country to renew her visa, which was never granted. Maria, whose birthday it had been when Pete died, had received the bad news (via email) that her father in Spain had died on the same day. She agonised about which funeral to go to, not wanting to miss either. She managed to carry on with her job, but found life difficult. Maria became the home manager after Ramesh. She stayed to support Maureen through her final illness and dying a year later, and to welcome new residents into the home during the following years.

Kathleen left two months after Pete's death. Her experience with Pete made her contemplate a return to nursing, with a focus on people with learning disabilities and end-of-life care. One support worker had joined the team only two weeks before Pete's death. She seemed relatively unaffected by it.

Services were not prepared for death

The men and women in the Veronica Project all needed increasing levels of physical support: more help with washing, dressing, using the toilet, moving about, taking medication. All this took time and called for extra staffing; without the support and commitment of senior management and social services to provide extra resources, the task of supporting a terminally ill resident at home became almost impossible.

The quality of support given to Lily, Pete, Dimas, Nick, Ursula, Ben and Marion in their residential care homes depended first of all on the willingness of the managers to take it on. But a simple willingness to provide extra staff was not enough; the staff also had to be willing to take on tasks they had not anticipated. As Stuart Todd points out, residential care services for people with learning disabilities were set up for the promotion of ordinary living, and may not be appropriate places for dying. 'A dying individual may prove an anomaly for staff... How well these staff are supported may well determine where the care of the dying takes place' (Todd 2002, p.233).

Some staff did not really want to support dying people. One support worker, whose own mother had recently died, said, 'I really don't want this to happen now.' Caring for a terminally ill resident meant not just an increase in physical demands; many support workers found themselves facing difficult emotions, other people's as well as their own, for which they were ill prepared.

Other researchers have described similar problems to the ones highlighted in the stories of Pete and Lily (Brown, Burns and Flynn 2002; Todd 2002). They spoke with carers in residential homes where someone with learning disabilities had died, and found that these homes were not prepared for the death. Communication and collaborative working with families and health care staff were lacking. There was insufficient recognition and support for the emotional involvement of staff. The carers didn't know whether and how to talk about dying. They were inexperienced and frightened: 'Please don't let it happen on my shift.'

Lack of resources and support

It was not so much clear service policies or structured support that made it possible for terminally ill residents to remain at home, but the willingness of committed staff members.

However, their dedication came at a cost. Several support workers were exhausted, and I sometimes worried that they were on the point of collapse or burn-out. This was particularly true for the home managers, who were acutely aware of their staff's need for support, but could not always get support for themselves. They were often ready to come in whenever there was a medical emergency, in the middle of the night if necessary. If there were gaps in staffing levels, they themselves often worked extra hours.

Extra support sometimes came from district nurses, who helped with medication or, in some cases, with washing and dressing. There are other support services available to cancer patients, for example, Marie Curie nurses who provide free care in patients' own homes, often at night. However, not all the residential services were aware of these potential sources of support. If they were, the need for extra support was not always anticipated in time. As a result, most of the extra demands had to be met by the support workers in the care home.

The effect of under-staffing was not only mental and physical exhaustion of support workers who were often desperate to give their resident the right support, but also inadequate care for the person who was ill. There was a further tension between trying to give the ill resident the necessary support, and coping with the ordinary needs of other residents. Ursula's home manager Mary said: 'It is hard because all the other residents need attention too, trying to give them a nice life, but we need so much time and attention for Ursula.'

It was not always easy for home managers to convince their superiors that extra staff was needed. When such support was put in place, it made all the difference, as we saw in Lily's case.

Mary and her husband ran an independent home. It was their business venture, and they themselves were responsible for negotiating extra resources with social services. It was a constant struggle for which Mary lacked the time and energy. When Ursula Smith was dying, she explained: 'I need one-to-one for her, really. Someone needs to be with her to feed her. She won't eat otherwise. It is a lot of work. I am almost begging the care manager, explaining it to him…'

When Ursula needed a wheelchair, Mary paid for one herself. 'You don't get things otherwise, you just have to go and organise it yourself. And Ursula really needed it. It is good, because now I can take her out.'

A year earlier, Mary had been deeply committed to Nick Ballard. She herself carried most of the burden, not only of care, but of cost. When his health deteriorated, she decided not to welcome a new resident into the only available downstairs bedroom, but converted the room for Nick instead, forgoing the extra money that would come from accepting a new resident.

The director of the care organisation that ran Ben Edwards' home reflected on the difficulties that occurred whenever Ben had to go into hospital. The home needed extra staff to enable someone to be with Ben and support him in an unfamiliar and sometimes frightening situation.

> 'We try to give the homes some extra support as soon as someone is diagnosed. It's difficult when people go into hospital, because social services won't pay for extra staff. They say it's not their responsibility, they're in the NHS now. We usually end up paying for it ourselves. It's difficult but we try to find the money somehow.'

Support workers are not health care staff

Health care professionals do not always recognise the fact that most staff in learning disability services are as inexperienced in looking after a dying person as ordinary families would be. At the same time as working on the Veronica Project, I carried out a survey of the experiences of palliative care staff working with people with learning disabilities (Tuffrey-Wijne *et al.* 2007b; Tuffrey-Wijne *et al.* 2008). There were several comments about the difficulty of getting generic health care services to provide the same level of care to people living in residential care homes as they would to ordinary patients living with their families. One hospice nurse said:

> 'We were trying to arrange for district nurses to come in to provide some more hands-on care because the staff at the home were not trained nurses. There was some reluctance from them to get involved. They very much felt that they shouldn't be going in to that kind of environment, because there were already staff there who should be doing it.'

Some carers in the Veronica Project complained that hospital staff didn't understand their role and expected them to continue providing their client with 24-hour care, even when they were admitted to hospital. Dimas Ferreira's support worker explained:

> 'It can be hard because we are not nurses, we are carers, but we are left to do the nursing with him. They don't always come

> into the room. I think they expect that they don't need to see to him, because we are here. But we are not nurses.'

Mary was furious at what she saw as the hospital's failure to look after Nick Ballard properly: 'The hospital expected us to stay with him, but I told them we couldn't, we don't have the staff, we have to support the other residents in the home.' She somehow coped when Ursula Smith was hospitalised:

> 'I sent in my staff, but I wasn't paid anything extra. So what I did was, I sent the morning staff straight to hospital, and when her shift ended there would be a one-hour gap before the next person came. My husband and I were just managing here at home.'

Inadequate facilities

The residential care homes in the Veronica Project typically opened in the 1970s and 1980s in response to the closure of long-stay hospitals. The philosophy was to enable people with learning disabilities to live lives in the community that were as 'normal' as possible. None of the residential care homes I visited was purpose-built. These were ordinary family homes in ordinary streets, that had been adapted to meet the needs of a group of three to eight residents. Some homes had a downstairs bedroom and bathroom, specially adapted for residents who were wheelchair users; but the bedrooms of the people in the Veronica Project were all upstairs. There were no lifts or stair lifts.

There were many recurring themes in the stories that make up the Veronica Project, but perhaps the most surprising was 'stairs'. It seemed so mundane and practical compared to the complexities of themes like truth-telling, family relationships and staff training, but stairs figured as an important issue for many people. Not being able to climb the stairs made life difficult for Lily, Pete, Nick, Ursula and Dimas. Ben and Marion remained able to manage the stairs, but their carers envisaged problems for them, too. Ben's home manager explained:

> 'We really want to keep him at home. I think that would be right. He loves his bedroom so much, I don't think he wants to move anywhere else. But we had the problem of a bed

downstairs for a while with someone else. He became really wobbly on his legs. The registration officer *[responsible for inspecting residential care homes]* didn't like him being down here.'

Dimas Ferreira died after a three-week hospital admission. There had been no plans about his place of death, but hospital certainly wasn't the preferred option. Dimas hated hospitals and was distressed during his final weeks. The hospice nurse who had supported the team in his home reflected afterwards:

> 'Had they been able to plan for his death, and where it would happen, I am not sure it would have been possible at home. His bedroom was upstairs, and it was very impractical, he wouldn't have been able to manage the stairs. He might have just stayed in his room, but I am not sure about that. I asked whether there was anywhere downstairs where he could have his bed, but it wasn't possible. There was one other person who had a bedroom downstairs, and it was not possible to swap.'

Families may well decide to move the bed of a beloved family member into the living room during the last weeks of life, but this is rarely an option for people who share their home with other people with learning disabilities. When individuals are too weak to manage the stairs, there are four available options: they move into a downstairs bedroom; they use a lift or stair lift; they become confined to their upstairs bedroom; or they move to a different care setting altogether. Clearly, the first two options need forward planning and resources. Such planning will become essential for learning disability services supporting an ageing population. Not many homes will be able to convert a downstairs room quickly for the benefit of a terminally ill resident, as Mary did for Nick Ballard. People's needs can change fast: Pete Carpenter climbed the stairs one week, but fell out of bed and couldn't manage those stairs the next.

Apart from the stairs, there were also problems about equipment and space. Not everyone dying of cancer needs bulky equipment, but some people needed a commode, a hoist, a wheelchair, a hospital bed. Even the most willing team will struggle to keep someone at home if the facilities are inadequate.

Support workers lack training and experience

One of the most striking aspects of Lily and Pete's stories is the inexperience of the support workers. The learning disability workforce in the UK is younger and less experienced than workers in other health and social care sectors. An estimated 75 per cent of the learning disability workforce is unqualified. Care workers have low status, and there are difficulties with recruitment and retention of care staff (Department of Health 2001a). Linda McEnhill writes:

> Despite this, many learning disability workers confront daily significant loss, emotional pain, and physical challenge... they receive little in the way of clinical supervision and due to budget restraints are not eligible for the vast range of educational opportunities. (McEnhill 2004, p.111)

Despite the best efforts of senior managers to give supervision and support, Lily and Pete's support workers felt uneasy. Other teams had similar insecurities: did they do the very best they could? Administering medication, in particular morphine, caused great anxiety. There was concern about picking up signs and symptoms that the cancer was getting worse. Support workers worried about 'missing something important'. They lacked the experience to know when someone entered the dying phase, and didn't always recognise the signs of impending death. The young support worker who sat with Pete as he drew his last breath didn't know that he had died until her colleague, who had more life experience, entered the room and realised; in the meantime, Ramesh was making a panicked phone call to the emergency services.

Ben Edwards' support workers faced a very similar situation when they found Ben on his bedroom floor in the early hours of the morning, breathing rapidly. They phoned Yanna, their manager, and an ambulance. When Yanna arrived, the ambulance crew was trying to resuscitate Ben. The support worker was physically shaking. She was young and had never seen anyone die. 'When I saw him lying on the floor, I thought he'd already gone,' said Yanna. Ben was taken to hospital and put on a life support machine, which was turned off later that day.

This contrasts sharply with the nurses at John Davies' nursing home: they had started giving him breakfast, but then realised that he was dying and simply sat with him.

Lack of knowledge was particularly hard for home managers, who were expected to explain the illness to other carers, including the family. Hospital staff were not always forthcoming with information. Yanna said:

> 'I need to talk to the family. But the doctors don't tell me everything. They only give me a little bit of information, and then they ask me to pass it on to the family... I need to know for myself, as well. I need to be able to plan things. I need to know what is happening.'

Although most support workers were inexperienced in health care matters, many had an intimate knowledge of the person they supported, without which it would be hard to notice the often subtle changes that indicate deteriorating health. However, their lack of status could make it difficult for them to act on this knowledge. Support workers who had no formal responsibilities for the home were least powerful and least able to challenge health professionals. When Marion Prentice was declared free of breast cancer, her 22-year-old support worker said:

> 'She is becoming more challenging again. I am just not happy. I don't know what to do about it. I tell the doctors, and they just think, "What does she know, she is not even trained." I tell them that this behaviour is not normal for Marion, that I think there is something wrong. She is more tired as well. But they just won't listen to me. Some people are saying, "She has Down's syndrome, she is old, it is just ageing." Well, maybe it is. Maybe I am just over-reacting. But I'm just not sure that the cancer is gone.'

Whether this support worker was correct could never be established, as symptoms of dementia took over. A year later, Marion was moved into a nursing home, away from the carers who knew her well. She died of heart failure.

The emotional impact of caring

Support workers in learning disability services can form close relationships with the people they care for. Such relationships are difficult to define. They are not family and they cannot take the family's place. However, many described themselves in such terms: 'We are like one big family'; 'He has nobody, so we are his family now.' Theirs was not just a job they could leave behind at the end of the day.

Of course, not all support workers are as dedicated. Lily's 15 years in the residential care home led her brother Bob to conclude:

> 'There are two types of carers in my mind. There are the ones who really care and are committed, and there are the ones for whom it is just a job. They often start with a lot of enthusiasm, they're going to do this and that, and then after a few months you find that they have left.'

Gary Butler, one of my research colleagues who has learning disabilities himself and who helped me to analyse the findings of the Veronica Project, lived in a staffed residential care home for nine years. He commented on my notes about Pete:

> 'The carers in that home seem really genuine. I found there's very few carers who are really genuine and supportive. Most of the staff don't really care, they're just there for the money. You know the difference when they are there when you need them. Some just say "I'm busy," they can't be bothered, and if I want to get something off my chest they don't listen.'

The people in the Veronica Project were maybe fortunate that they had the support of such 'genuine' carers. However, the emotional impact of caring – really caring – for a person with learning disabilities who was ill and dying was considerable. It was not unusual for support workers to be on the verge of tears when I talked to them about their own needs or showed concern for them. They invoked the memories of their own family members who had died, or of another ill and dying resident they had cared for in the past. They realised that they were not family, really; but they sometimes resembled family members in the way the ill or dying person dominated their lives and emotions. It kept them awake at night.

When Dimas Ferreira was dying in hospital, he was visited by a support worker who had been on maternity leave. She hadn't seen him for several months. She took one look at the pale and thin man lying unconscious among the white sheets, and put her hand to her mouth in shock. She left the room for a moment, crying. Dimas' aunt was moved by this: 'I always felt they love him. It is not a show they put on for me. You saw her reaction. It means a lot to me.'

Another of Dimas' support workers was sitting at his bedside, holding his hand, and explained:

> 'It is hard for me and my colleagues, really hard. I thought he was going to die yesterday, he looked so awful. I am doing nursing training and I have worked with elderly people, so I have been at death beds before. That is not so difficult for me. But some of my colleagues can't cope with it. They don't want to see him, they find it too hard at the moment. We take it in turns to be here, with the staff who can cope. I would have liked him to be at home, but we can't do nursing. Like this morning, he needed extra injections of morphine, and we can't do that. That's why he needs to be here.'

Close bonds

People with learning disabilities are among the most vulnerable and dependent people in society. Their dependency had an impact on the support workers. Whilst there are many short-term members of staff and agency staff working in learning disability services, there are also considerable numbers of support workers who have known their clients for years. One such support worker said, 'You do get attached to them. You can't help it.'

Here is someone whom they help to wash and dress, take to the toilet, help to eat; someone whose communication they have learned to interpret; someone who relies on them. People with learning disabilities, particularly those who so clearly need their carers, can call forth a huge amount of compassion and involvement. Carers can become fiercely protective when the person they look after becomes seriously ill.

Many carers went well beyond the call of duty. Dimas Ferreira's support worker said, 'I would do anything for him. Anything. I come in on my days off, I don't mind. He is such a lovely person.' Similarly, the support workers for Pete, Lily, Marion and Ben worked many unpaid extra hours, accompanying them to important hospital appointments even if it wasn't their shift, and visiting them on their days off.

Mary used similar words: 'I love Nick to bits, I would do anything.' She was available to him 24 hours a day, taking her young daughters with her if needed, and she was prepared to forgo her holidays for his sake. The urge to be available at all times was magnified by the sense that there was no one else who could provide the same kind of support. Mary said: 'Even if I had more staff, or more experienced staff, I would still want to do it all myself. Because I know the person, and care for them, and that is my job.'

The close emotional bonds between people with learning disabilities and their support workers are important. Ben Edwards' brother commented: 'Yanna is like a mother to him. She really is. Whenever Ben is not happy or well he always asks for Yanna. She is always there for him.'

Sometimes, I saw that carers patronised adults with learning disabilities and treated them like children. It is of course important that carers respect those they care for; but what seemed even more important to the people in the Veronica Project was that their carers showed genuine affection. They needed warmth and empathy. There was no substitute for love. Carers like Mary and Yanna were hugely important in people's lives; they were sensitive to their needs, and they provided them with safety and support.

But the emotional bonds meant that the carers were vulnerable themselves. The deterioration and dying of the people they cared for could be utterly devastating. Rules, regulations and shift patterns were almost irrelevant; support workers who had made an emotional investment needed to be supported. Even those who were not particularly close to the ill person could be emotionally fragile because of the confrontation with death. Their need for support was under-estimated by senior managers and by outside services, such as GPs, hospice teams or community learning disability teams.

There is no easy way to accompany another human being on his or her journey towards death. The carers were bound to grieve when the person died, but they were surprised by the strength of their grief. They knew they cared deeply, yet they also saw themselves as professionals who should be able to cope. Their grief was disenfranchised (Doka 1989): they did not see themselves, and were not recognised by others, as people who had lost a loved one.

Supporting the carers

Home managers were crucial in the support of people with learning disabilities who were seriously ill. They acted as role models, leading their teams in their commitment to support the ill resident; it also fell to them to support their team members and to negotiate for extra resources with senior managers in the organisation. How much support the senior managers were actually able to give to the home manager, practical as well as emotional, had a major impact on all the staff and on the dying person. How well the home managers were supervised and supported by these senior managers had a great impact on the care they were able to give.

A few days after Ben Edwards died, Yanna was thinking about her staff team and possible ways in which she could support them. She felt supported herself. 'The area manager has been ringing me,' she said appreciatively. 'She rang again today.'

Things were much more difficult for Mary, who owned and ran an independent home. She did not have a line manager or a peer group of other managers. It was hard for her to see social services as a source of support because she was so often fighting them for resources, and because they had the power to close down her business if it did not meet their standards.

Home managers are not always aware of the kind of support available from outside services. Community learning disability teams or hospice teams, for example, are less likely to become involved if the homes don't ask for their help. The hospice nurse involved in Nick Ballard's care thought that Mary was coping well, and didn't visit unless she was asked – but Mary was unaware of the potential support this nurse could give, and didn't think she needed any advice.

It was easier if home managers felt able to delegate the exhausting business of round-the-clock support to their staff, and share the load. Marion Prentice's team found particularly effective ways of sharing out the various tasks. It was Marion's key worker who did most of the planning and support for Marion, prepared her for hospital appointments, liaised with her doctors and her sister. The key worker herself received intensive supervision and support from the home manager, relieving not only the physical burden but also the emotional strain. The home manager sometimes made a point of asking other support workers to be with Marion in hospital, because she was concerned that Marion would otherwise associate her key worker too much with hospitals and illness.

What the carers seemed to need was a trusted outside professional who was fully available to them, with whom they could discuss their worries, and who knew where to get practical and emotional support for the team. There were such professionals around, doctors or nurses willing to provide support, but the support workers often felt they could not possibly make demands on their precious time. Maybe later, maybe once things got really bad… As a researcher who visited regularly, who was interested in everything that happened, and who was also seen as someone with experience and understanding of the issues involved, I became a sounding board for many of the families and paid carers in the Veronica Project. This was particularly poignant for carers who did not have any other support. Once, when I turned up at Ursula Smith's home, Mary opened the door, looking exhausted. I put my arm around her, acknowledging the difficult time she was having, and she said, 'Oh my god, I'm glad to see you. I'm telling you, I've been so stressed. It's just all too much.'

Teams that were coping on their own were not only at risk of collapse; the lack of outside support was also detrimental to the care of the person with learning disabilities.

Health care professionals

People with cancer spend a lot of time in hospitals, and many move to a health care setting at the end of life. Only three people in the Veronica Project died at home, two of which were residential care homes for people with learning disabilities; seven people died in a hospital, hospice or nursing home. We will focus here on people's encounters with health care staff, as this influenced their experience of cancer and dying.

During the latter half of the Veronica Project, the health care of people with learning disabilities was in the national news several times. Mencap published a report called *Death by Indifference*, describing the deaths of six people with learning disabilities in hospitals and claiming that those deaths were the result of institutional discrimination (Mencap 2007). Investigating these allegations, the Health Ombudsman found that in four of the six cases the person concerned was treated less favourably for reasons related to his or her learning disabilities; at least one person died as a direct result of an unacceptable standard of care and treatment (Parliamentary and Health Service Ombudsman 2009). An independent inquiry into access to health care for people with learning disabilities found convincing evidence that people with learning disabilities have higher levels of unmet need and receive less effective treatment. It said:

> There is insufficient attention given to making reasonable adjustments to support the delivery of equal treatment, as required by the Disability Discrimination Act. Adjustments are not always made to allow for communication problems, difficulty in understanding (cognitive impairment), or the anxieties and preferences of individuals concerning their treatment. (Michael 2008, p.7)

How did the experiences of the 13 people in the Veronica Project compare with these rather shocking reports?

One sensitive health care professional could make a difference

One positive finding was that a single dedicated and sensitive doctor or nurse could transform someone's experience. There were examples of exemplary practice. John Davies was supported throughout his illness by a wonderfully caring Macmillan cancer nurse at the hospital, who tried hard to understand his needs and those of his family. John trusted her and looked out for her. Vincent Sweeney came to rely on his hospice nurse, who took an interest in him, as a source of support – he was very upset when she later took him off her caseload. Lily Lamb's hospice nurses took the time to get to know her, to understand her communication and work out what she needed.

However, having sensitive doctors and nurses seemed to be a matter of luck. As the government's independent inquiry found: 'For the most part, innovation and good practice owes more to the enthusiasm of energetic individuals than to any structured and systematic engagement by health services' (Michael 2008, p.9).

Unfortunately, insensitive staff could have the opposite effect. Marion Prentice's support worker described a doctor who needed to drain some fluid from Marion's breast.

> 'He approached her, without saying anything to her, and I thought he was just going to feel her chest. But he suddenly came with this huge needle, and an enormous syringe attached to that, and he just stuck it in and pulled the syringe. She was screaming, she was in agony. She was in such a state. He asked me to hold her down. It was just awful. And then finally he took it out and said, "Oh well, that didn't work"... She was really frightened of doctors after that. We had to go home, we couldn't do anything else with her. And when we came back another day, we specially requested to see a different doctor. The one we saw then was really nice. He talked to her and told her what he was going to do. He had a very small syringe, and put it in and just drained all the fluid out. It didn't hurt her at all.'

I asked this support worker what made the difference between Marion being scared and uncooperative, and Marion being fine. She replied:

> 'It's the way people talk to her. If you just look at her, and talk to her, shake her hand: she loves that. Just tell her what is going on. Include her. But if you simply talk to me without looking at her, and do things to her without warning: forget it. It's not difficult, really.'

Being ignored

It can be difficult for doctors and nurses with little experience of learning disability to know how to include someone with cognitive limitations or limited speech in the conversation. They often needed the carers to help them out. It was easiest, least uncomfortable, when they acknowledged this limitation openly.

The hospice nurse who came to assess Pete Carpenter at home spent a few minutes chatting to him about the cycling magazine he showed her. When she needed to move on and find out more about his background, she said to Ramesh, 'I don't quite know how to do this bit. Does Pete mind us talking about him like this?' I helped them out: 'Pete, is it OK if the nurse talks to Ramesh about you?' Pete was fine; he liked the nurse, and the attention she showed him seemed to make him feel included.

The radiographer carrying out Marion's mammogram spoke to Marion first, but realised that she did not get the right answers to her questions ('Do you know your birthday?' 'Yes.' 'When is it?' 'Yes.') Addressing the support worker instead, the radiographer said how uncomfortable she felt, talking over people's heads.

In fact, it was not the 'talking over people's heads' in itself that excluded them; it was the way in which this was done. It was inevitable that some of the information had to be obtained from the carers. Health workers who did acknowledge the person with learning disabilities, like those quoted above, were able to build up a positive and supportive relationship. This could be as simple as greeting someone with learning disabilities.

Ben Edwards liked his hospital appointments, not only because of the videos he could buy in the shop, but also because the nurses knew him and talked to him. Hospice staff were particularly good at treating people with respect. Here is what happened during Sally Burnett's first days in the hospice.

> *When someone comes into the room (domestic staff, nursing assistant, physiotherapist), even when they do not come particularly for Sally, they invariably smile at her and greet her. Most look at me first, but when they talk to us, they address Sally first. The social worker comes in briefly, just to say hello. She is continually focused on Sally, and asks her, 'Who is this? Is this your friend?' 'Yes,' says Sally. 'Will you introduce me?' asks the social worker. She needs to repeat this a few times before Sally understands, but doesn't give up. 'This is Irene,' Sally says eventually.*

This contrasted sharply with our experience in hospital the week before. Sitting at people's bedside in hospital, I found that they were hardly ever spoken to by the hospital staff; the following description of the doctors' round for Sally exemplified this.

> *They stand at the end of the bed; the doctors read through the notes, with the nurse simply waiting, looking on. None of them look at Sally or acknowledge her. Occasionally, they look at me, but nobody introduces him- or herself, or asks me who I am... Sally just keeps staring rather blankly, at a doctor*

(nobody looks back), at a curtain rail, at me (giving me a smile, the only emotion she shows). Sometimes, her eyes droop. She is quite sleepy. [The four doctors spend several minutes debating Sally's medical condition.]

It is only when one of the doctors needs to examine Sally that he starts talking to her. He is quite friendly, and Sally responds. The trouble is that she nods or says 'yes' to all his questions, even if I know it to be 'no': Have you been sick? Have you eaten anything? Are you OK? Do you feel nauseous? Yes, yes, yes, yes.

I stay for the physical examination. The doctor palpates her abdomen. She simply sits through it. He then tells her, speaking quickly and with a strong accent, that she will be able to eat again once she feels less nauseous, just see how it goes, try a little bit, etc etc, is that OK? 'Yes,' she says in a strong voice, but I know that she doesn't have a clue what he talked about. She probably couldn't even hear him properly. Afterwards, they all troop out. Nobody says goodbye to her or even acknowledges her. They simply walk away.

It may be that such doctors' rounds are not unusual, and that patients without learning disabilities also experience a lack of engagement or courtesy from some doctors. What surprised me was that whilst I was invariably shocked at the insensitivity of doctors and nurses, the people with learning disabilities simply seemed to accept it. It was as if they were used to not being spoken to.

Once, when Pete Carpenter was in hospital, a nurse came in and stood behind him. She said something about his mouth being dirty and wiped the inside of his mouth clean with a cloth, all the time standing behind him, not addressing him and not looking him in the eye. I felt outraged, but Pete was gracious and resigned.

Not understanding what is happening

There were a number of incidents where the people with learning disabilities were taken by surprise; incidents that were upsetting and that could easily have been prevented by simple explanations. The draining of Marion's breast was one such example. Other incidents were less dramatic, but added to the people's bewilderment or distress. This is what happened to Ben Edwards and his bag.

The ward sister turns up with another nurse, telling me: 'I'm sorry, we have to move his bed to another bay… We'll put him somewhere nice and quiet,

> *so you can carry on talking.' The bed is wheeled out. They tell him that they are going to move his bed to another bay, and he nods: 'Yeah.' I am not at all sure he has understood, so I tell him, using sign language: 'You're going to a new room.' 'Yes,' he says. But when they come back to wheel out his bedside cabinet, with his full bag on top, he gets upset: 'My bag!' He gets up, grabs hold of the bag.*
>
> *'No, let go, we are going to move it,' says the nurse. 'We are moving it to another bay.' They take it off him, put it back on the locker, and wheel it out. Ben looks at it going, alarmed. 'My bag! Going home!' he says. There is confusion on his face. He clearly hasn't understood about the moving bed. 'Come, let's go and find the bag,' I say, and offer him my arm. He takes it, relieved, and off we go.*

The nurses were probably unaware of the distress this episode had caused. Ben's understanding of spoken words was limited; what he needed was someone to show him where his bed was going, someone to take him along with the bag.

Hospitals could be difficult places for people who weren't sure what was happening. Even if someone was willing to come along for an appointment, waiting times could be a challenge. 'Taxi,' Pete Carpenter said anxiously as the waiting took too long – he wanted to go home, and couldn't understand why he had to sit in the waiting room for over an hour.

The challenge of communication

Hospital staff often seemed nervous and unsure around people with learning disabilities. Here is Ben Edwards again.

> *Ben says to the nurses, loudly: 'Go home!' He wants to go home. He had already asked me, and after a while I'd figured out what he was saying: 'Ambulance.' He meant that he wanted to take an ambulance home.*
>
> *The nurses look at each other and laugh. He is saying he wants to go home! 'Not today,' says one of them, laughing. Ben looks at her with a question mark in his eyes. He is not sure what she is saying.*
>
> *He asks me again, but I have already said that I don't know, and he repeats that now. 'Don't know?'*

The nurses left me to it. It was not the only time that I was left to explain things, to act as a bridge between the hospital staff and their patient. When I left soon afterwards, Ben's nurse asked me with some alarm, 'Are you going?!'

Staff in hospitals and hospices were unaware of the range of communication techniques that could be useful for people with learning disabilities. They relied heavily on spoken words, often using complex sentences, even at times when simply showing what was happening would have been easier and more effective: holding up a syringe or a mouth wipe; showing someone his or her new room. Mary, who was expected by hospital staff to be with Nick Ballard constantly during his admissions, explained how different things were at another hospital, where Nick was once admitted as an emergency.

> 'They had this picture board for people who had had strokes. It was wonderful. It had pictures of all the things you might need: pyjamas, slippers, tea, everything. Nick would just point to what he wanted. He would point at pyjamas and they would bring him some. I didn't have to be there all the time, because he could communicate that way. I haven't seen anything like that here.'

Ursula Smith's hospital nurse explained to me how hard it was to look after someone with severe communication difficulties. Ursula had come into hospital and died the next day. Her nurse reflected afterwards:

> 'It was difficult to understand her. We couldn't understand what she wanted. But then she shouted, "Water, water, water," and we could understand that. I have looked after other patients with learning disabilities before, but they have stayed longer, two or three weeks. So then you get used to how they speak, and it is easier… I think she was anxious. She was shouting a lot. I don't think she liked being here. She wanted to be at home. We talked about sending her back home, but we didn't really have time to organise it. We had so little time.'

Sally tended to answer 'yes' to whatever question the doctor asked her, even if the truthful answer was 'no'. Many people with learning disabilities have a tendency to agree with the questioner, regardless of the question. Some try to hide the fact that they don't know the answer to a question. When Pete's doctor asked him: 'How old are you, Mr Carpenter?' he answered convincingly and without hesitation: 'Twenty-eight'.

Health care staff seemed mostly unaware of such communication characteristics of some people with learning disabilities, or maybe they did not know how to adapt their own way of communicating in order to meet the person's needs. This could make assessment very difficult for doctors and nurses (Tuffrey-Wijne and McEnhill 2008).

Communication difficulties were frustrating for both people with learning disabilities and staff. Relatives and support workers were often very good at understanding what the person wanted, but in their absence, things could be difficult. This is illustrated by the following episode at Lily Lamb's hospice:

> *Just before the nurses leave Lily, she says something that sounds to me like 'arm'. The nurse, too, thinks Lily is talking about pain in her arm. Lily is getting slightly frustrated, and starts pointing to the wall, making a squeezing gesture with her hand. I think she is pointing at the medicine cupboard, and ask her whether she is talking about the painkillers that get sprayed into her mouth sometimes. She keeps saying 'arm', pointing and squeezing, until finally it dawns on me and the nurse that she wants the call buzzer ('alarm') which is also on the wall, next to the medicine cabinet. I feel frustrated for her. Once I know what she means, it seems blindingly obvious: the words, the pointing, the miming. It is us, me and the nurse, who have the problem, not understanding.*

Ignorance

I did not find any evidence of intentionally unkind or uncaring health care staff. Most doctors and nurses are compassionate and want to do the best for their patients, including patients with learning disabilities. But to build effective therapeutic relationships with people with learning disabilities, health care professionals have to come out of their comfort zone. They have to communicate in unusual ways; they have to stop and find a way to connect, even if it is just with eye contact.

Some health care staff made that effort. I felt that the failure of many others was not due to ill will, and not to lack of time, but to ignorance and fear.

Summary

Services were not prepared for death

- The ability of residential care homes to support a terminally ill resident depended on the willingness and commitment of the home managers.
- Residential care homes often had inadequate staffing levels to cope with the increased care needs of a terminally ill resident. Most of the extra demands were met by over-stretched support workers. Support from outside agencies was not always organised in time. Home managers struggled to negotiate extra resources with their senior management or social services.
- Facilities in residential care homes were inadequate. The fact that bedrooms were upstairs, with no lift or stair lift, was problematic in all residential care homes.
- Support workers are not medically trained, and are highly inexperienced in looking after a terminally ill resident. They felt unsure and often very anxious, particularly about giving medication and about death.
- Outside professionals often did not realise that the support workers were inexperienced, and expected them to cope with the new physical care needs.
- Many support workers had formed close emotional bonds with their clients. They went well beyond the call of duty, working extra hours or coming in on days off. They were vulnerable to feelings of distress and loss. This was not always recognised and supported by managers.
- Support workers needed emotional support themselves. Home managers were particularly vulnerable. They did their best to support their teams, but did not always ask for or receive support for themselves.

Inexperienced health care professionals

- There were some highly sensitive nurses and doctors who took an interest in their patient and tried to understand their needs. This could transform the person's experience. However, there was no systematic engagement with people with learning disabilities by health care services: having sensitive health care professionals was 'luck of the draw'.
- Many health care staff ignored the person with learning disabilities and related exclusively to the carers. Some instigated procedures without explanation or warning.
- Health care staff were nervous and unsure about communicating with people with learning disabilities. They were unaware of specific communication characteristics (e.g. the tendency to agree with the questioner), or of the range of possible communication techniques.
- Lack of sensitive care was not due to ill will, but to ignorance and fear among health care staff.

CHAPTER 6

Dependent Lives

Were the experiences of the people in the Veronica Project unique to people with learning disabilities who have cancer? Would they happen to all people with learning disabilities? Would they happen to all people with cancer? It was not always easy to answer these questions. There was no control group. The aim of the Veronica Project was simply to try to understand people's worlds.

Yet, as the study progressed, what struck me more than anything was the way in which people's life stories affected the stories of their cancer and their dying. In order to understand what it was like for them to be dying of cancer, I had to try to understand what their lives had been like. This is, of course, true for all dying people. Our family bonds, the relationships we have built, the things we have done, the culture we come from, our place in the world, our self-image, will all affect the way in which we will experience the losses that come with dying. What struck me in the Veronica Project was how different the lives of the participants had been from the lives of most of us. Sometimes it was very hard to imagine what their lives had been like at all; when I tried, it could be painful even to think about it. The 13 life stories were very different from each other, but there was a common thread that defined them, and that ultimately defined people's experience of illness and dying.

What the people in the Veronica Project had in common was 'dependence'. They had been dependent on others throughout their lives in ways few of the rest of the adult population are. All of their lives had somehow been deprived: there was bullying and abuse, lack of relationships, lack of choice, lack of stimulation, and a lifelong experience of being less important than others. How such life experiences impacted on the experience of illness and dying is the focus of this chapter.

The story of Lily Lamb's life

Lily and her older brother Bob were born in London, where Lily attended a school for children with special needs. The school suited her. It was devastating for her when the family had to move to Cornwall, where no such facilities were available. The local authority insisted that Lily should have some kind of schooling, and she was sent to a mainstream school. It was not a happy time. Lily sat at the back of the class and couldn't keep up with her classmates, who made fun of her. She came home crying every day. After a year her desperate parents took the only other option, again on the advice of the local authority, and sent her to a special needs boarding school some distance away. No visits were allowed for the first month. Bob remembered how he would sometimes go and see Lily with his parents, and there would be more tears. Lily stayed at the boarding school for several unhappy years until the family moved back to London, partly to make Lily's life easier. She was now 16 years old.

Lily started attending day care facilities, and throughout the following decades she was offered various activities and classes. 'The thing is,' said Bob, 'they always did the same things! She would be offered a course, and it would be one of four things, and it never changed. She was really bored and fed up. So I couldn't believe it when her appraisal would come round at the home, and they would talk about what she might want to do, and they suggested that she could do a course in silk painting… she'd go, "NO!" and we'd go, "Oh no, not another course of silk painting, she's done that so many times."'

Lily loved to do things well. She loved proper work and was delighted when she could start packing airline cutlery, getting paid a little bit of money at the end of the week. She was proud of the fact that she did a good job, never packing two spoons and no knife. It never bored her. She hated it when the packing was abolished (Bob remembered talk of exploitation and the use of politically incorrect labour), and she went back to dancing and silk painting. Later, the organisation that ran her residential home offered her work in their office, and she set off proudly each morning to spend some happy hours shredding papers.

Lily did not make any real friends in her life. At her residential home and day centre, she related almost exclusively to the staff and carers. Maybe she would have liked to have friends, but she was always rather self-conscious about not being able to speak properly and being overweight. When she was at the hospice, Lily enjoyed the many people who popped into her room: nurses, therapists, volunteers. 'She has never been so popular in her life!' May commented. 'Never. She hasn't really had anyone in her life who took an interest in her, apart from her mum and dad, Bob and myself. And she was always quite unsociable, insecure maybe. She wouldn't just talk to people. But in here, she has been talking to everyone.'

Deprivation and dependence

Bullying and abuse

Once I realised that I had to find out about people's lives as well as their final illness, I stopped focusing explicitly on 'cancer'. I told the men and women that I was interested in everything: not only their illness, their experiences of doctors and nurses and hospitals, but also their childhoods, their families, the things they had done in their life, the things they had enjoyed, the things that had been hard. Almost without exception, those who could tell me chose to start by talking of their childhood experiences, and what they spoke of first of all was their experience of being bullied, of not being part of things, maybe even of being abused.

- *John Davies*: 'Name calling…it's the worst thing that happens, and it's not a picnic being called a spastic.'
- *Vincent Sweeney*: 'When I was about 15 or 16, I was [sexually] abused… I never told anyone.'
- *Richard Horwood*: 'I was bullied at school. There were other boys, ten years old, and they would bully me and beat me. I

would come home with a black eye and bruises. They knew I wouldn't do anything back, that's why they could do it.'

- *Richard's sister*: 'It wasn't just the other children, you know. He would come home with his pockets sewn up so he couldn't put his hands in them... I was worried when he came here *[living in his own flat]*. He is so vulnerable.'

I didn't ask people about bullying or abuse, but I discovered that all 13 men and women had experienced bullying. Those who could speak told me about it; the families of those who couldn't speak painted a similar picture. As children, they had endured playground taunts or were laughed at for not going to a 'normal' school. Vincent Sweeney remembered how much it hurt to be called 'dim'.

Other abuse could only be guessed at. No one knew why Dimas Ferreira's nose was as crooked as it was, having been broken several times somewhere in his past. Ben Edwards often talked about being hit: 'Cliff Richard hit me,' he said, banging on his chest. Four of the people who had lived in long-stay hospitals had all their teeth removed when they were young, presumably as a precaution against biting.

As adults, people remained vulnerable to bullying and abuse. They were sometimes angry, sometimes resigned to this. Richard Horwood and Charlie, the friend he shared his house with, were regularly hassled by local children. Richard said, with a shrug of his shoulders: 'I don't think they mean any harm, they're just kids. Charlie and I have learning disabilities, that's why they do it.'

Sally Burnett's stepmother Joy didn't think Sally had been bullied. Sally was the only person for whom this issue had not emerged, so I had asked Joy about it. But it may be that some bullying was, as in Richard's case, simply taken for granted. Joy later remembered:

> 'One day I came home and I noticed that the glass had gone from her dad's picture. I had his photograph in a frame in the room. I said to her, "Where's the glass gone?" And she said, "I threw my slipper at it." I said, "What'd you do that for?" She said it was because people in the bus had made fun of her... Sometimes I noticed it in her flat as well. There would be a few dents in the wall, and I'd say, "What's happened there?" and she'd say that she had thrown something.'

This experience of being bullied and abused, going right back to childhood, had coloured people's lives. It affected their perception of themselves and of their place in life.

People's dependence on others made them vulnerable. This was most painfully evident in the case of Ursula Smith. I will describe in some detail what happened during one of my visits, because it illustrates just how vulnerable people with learning disabilities can be, even in adulthood, right up to their final illness.

Ursula Smith: an incident of abuse

Helena, an untrained support worker in her late thirties, had worked at Ursula's home ever since Ursula had arrived from a long-stay hospital 18 years ago. She had always refused to attend training sessions, arguing that her many years of experience were sufficient. Mary, the home manager, had not forced her; Helena was her only long-term member of staff, and Mary relied on her.

Ursula had long-standing mental health problems and had been on medication for bipolar disorder for longer than anyone remembered. I didn't know her well. This was my second visit, and she was very weak (although nobody realised quite how weak: she died three weeks later). She was sitting in the armchair by her bed, a small hunched-up figure, hiding her face, her nose almost touching her lap. Helena had brought us each a mug of coffee, and now the two of us were just sitting together, mostly in silence. This is where my notes pick up the story.

> *Once, I ask her whether she wants her coffee. It is cool enough to drink now. She looks up from her doziness, says a loud 'No' and puts her head back on her chest straight away. 'OK,' I say.*
>
> *Helena comes in. She shakes Ursula. 'Ursula, drink your coffee now. It will be cold.' She picks up the coffee, puts it to Ursula's lips.*
>
> *'No!' says Ursula very loudly. She puts her head on her chest and closes her eyes. 'No, come on Ursula, you're not sleepy, you've got to drink it,' says Helena, keeping the mug firmly to Ursula's mouth, taking her by the back of her head with her other hand. 'No! I don't want it!' says Ursula, pushing the drink away.*
>
> *What ensues leaves me in utter turmoil. Helena keeps telling Ursula that she has to drink the coffee and forces it down her throat. Ursula is trying to*

push it away, putting her hand over the cup, spilling some of it. Helena has a firm grip of both Ursula's head and the mug, and keeps tipping some of it into Ursula's mouth. 'Come on, you have to drink it.'

I say weakly, 'You don't want that drink, do you, Ursula?' Helena keeps looking at me intermittently, smiling conspiratorially, saying, 'This is what we've got to do, she wouldn't drink anything otherwise.' And to Ursula: 'The doctor says you've got to drink. You want to go to hospital? If you don't drink, we can't keep you here.'

By the time the mug is empty (and Helena insists on her drinking it to the very last drop) Ursula is shouting and lashing out. She is crying at the same time. Frankly, I don't blame her. I want to kick the coffee away myself. I want to cry. I am completely appalled. 'Abuse' is the term that keeps going through my head. What can I do? What should I do?... I find it almost impossible to witness what seems to me bullying, even abusive behaviour. I know it is all meant in the best of ways; I know Helena cares about Ursula; and yet...

'Right, now you need to go to the toilet,' says Helena. 'No,' shouts Ursula. 'Yes, you have to,' says Helena. I get out of the way, sitting down on Ursula's bed. Helena manhandles Ursula out of her chair, putting her hand under Ursula's armpit and hoiking her up. Ursula soon gives in, and they walk out of the room... I am struck by how thin she is. A small, hunched-up torso on very thin legs. Her clothes hanging off her.

When they are away on the toilet, I sit on the bed feeling utterly distressed. I am almost in tears. I want to shout and lash out, too.

When they come back, and Ursula sits down again, a tear plops onto her oversized bib. Helena pinches Ursula's cheek, holding it firmly. 'See, she is depressed.'

She leaves. Thank goodness. I can't bear it. If I were crying, would I want to have my cheek pinched? Definitely not. I would want someone to come and sit with me, and acknowledge how hard things are. They don't have to stop my tears. They have to be able to sit through them. All this jolliness. 'Do this, do that'...

I go back to Ursula, sitting down as closely as I can. I put my hand on her arm. 'Oh, Ursula,' I say. 'I didn't know your life is so hard. You really didn't want to drink that coffee, and you had to drink it. And then you didn't want to get up and go to the toilet.' The tears drip onto the bib, plop-plop. 'I wanted to find out what your life is like, and now I can see that it is hard. You were shouting, and now you are crying...'

She lifts up her head and looks at me. She turns her face back to her lap. And she sobs. The tears flow and flow. Large drips of snot hang off her nose.

> *'It's OK, Ursula,' I tell her. 'I don't mind if you cry. It is good to cry when you are sad. And I can see that you are sad.'*
>
> *For the next 20 minutes, we sit like this. She cries. I make quiet noises, just saying the occasional word: 'Oh dear, Ursula...' Every time I say something like that, the crying that had reduced to the occasional teardrop is a renewed sobbing.*
>
> *I don't know what the crying means. To start with, she sobs a few loud sentences, but I cannot make out any of the words. There is Sally [Burnett] in my mind: 'Oh, yes, she is always crying,' people around Sally would say, almost dismissively. It is probably the same for Ursula. I have already been told this. She is always crying. There is a sense of 'never mind, nothing to be done' behind this. But for me, the crying is new. The distress is new. And sitting next to Ursula, I can feel it inside me. I am quivering inside, and it would be quite easy for me to sit and cry with her.*
>
> *Eventually, Ursula stops crying. She slowly quietens, and eventually her eyes are closed again, and her breathing returns to dozing. After five minutes of this, I tell her: 'I am going now, Ursula. It was lovely to see you. I enjoyed sitting with you. I know you were sad, but it doesn't matter. I liked being with you.' I ask her: 'Can I come and see you again next week?' At this point she looks up at me, and says a very clear 'Yes'.*

Afterwards, I was upset with myself for not intervening; but I was taken aback by the openness with which Helena forced Ursula to drink her coffee. I needed to talk to members of the research advisory group in order to clarify my role as a researcher. My view that Helena's behaviour constituted abuse was vindicated. When I reported it to Mary and it was investigated by social services, Helena was suspended and subsequently left her job.

Not all Ursula's carers were as controlling and forceful as Helena. I had seen how Mary herself spent long periods of time with Ursula, gently and lovingly encouraging her to eat and drink; Ursula was perfectly capable of feeding herself if she wanted to. But support workers have considerable power over vulnerable residents, and the abuse of such power can be damaging. The effects can go unnoticed.

One of the shocking aspects of the situation was that neither Ursula nor Helena regarded the incident as abusive. During the investigations, Ursula denied that anyone had ever hurt her, saying 'Helena looks after me!' Helena herself may even have thought that she demonstrated good care, showing me how she ensured that Ursula drank enough.

People with learning disabilities have often led difficult lives, and it is not always easy to support them. Their behaviour can be challenging. The residents in Ursula's home sometimes screamed and shouted, cried loudly, or destroyed things. To support people who are upset or angry requires maturity and self-awareness. It is easy to see how support workers themselves can become impatient or even rough. When people with learning disabilities become ill, and the demands increase, they are even more at risk.

Like Helena, the people who support them are often poorly paid, poorly trained, poorly supervised – as well as over-worked and tired. Such staff are under-valued by society, and maybe society expects too much from them. Maybe what was surprising in the Veronica Project was not that some support workers abused their power over vulnerable residents, but that there were so many support workers who were able to provide mature and sensitive support.

Lack of a sexual identity

The many limitations of people's lives included a lack of loving relationships with partners. They were often not perceived as adults with a sexual identity. Times may be changing, and nowadays sexual relationships are less frowned upon, particularly for people with mild learning disabilities; but for the people in the Veronica Project, forming attachments with partners that were openly acknowledged by the people around them had not been possible. Only Amanda Cresswell, who was in her thirties and had recovered from cancer, had a boyfriend who was accepted as such by family and friends. Vincent Sweeney lamented: 'I would really like a girlfriend, but I can't have a relationship... I have nothing.' John Davies kept the nature of any intimate relationships he may have had in his life private, but acknowledged the sadness of losing 'the chance of any kind of relationship with anybody' that his illness had brought. Once, he said: 'Sometimes I think, I wish I could have had children. You know? I sometimes sit there and think, who is going to look after me when I get old and grey?'

John Davies' hospice staff was impressively insightful and reflective. After his death, they called a meeting to discuss the support of people with learning disabilities. What could they learn from their involvement with John? One staff member pondered regretfully:

> 'I never discussed sexuality with him. I know it is difficult with most patients, but with anyone else I would have picked it up, I would have opened up a conversation about sexuality. Why didn't I with John? I think it was him having learning disabilities that stopped me.'

There was a lack of acceptance of the people with learning disabilities as sexual beings, and sometimes their sexuality was openly mocked. One support worker spoke indulgently of a man's interest in another resident's visiting relative: 'She has long blonde hair, and he will go to her and take her hand. Oh, he has an eye for the ladies, that one. I tell him, "Are you chatting her up?!" and it makes him laugh.'

It was a lifelong sadness, the difficulty of finding and sustaining loving relationships with partners that could be accepted and supported by the outside world, the absence of children of your own; and it was people's deteriorating health, the way this made them reflect on their lives, that brought out keen feelings of loss. One wonderfully caring and perceptive support worker told me about David, a 54-year-old man with Down's syndrome who had lived in the home of Pete Carpenter and died a few years ago. David was a family man, someone who relished his relationships with his brothers, nieces and nephews. When he was dying, he was in turmoil. The support worker said:

> 'I think he was furious. He had always wanted to get married. He didn't have a girlfriend, but in his last days he said, "I thought that I would have been engaged." Now he realised it wasn't ever going to happen.'

Loneliness

One further effect of not having partners or children was that most people in the Veronica Project had no roles of real responsibility for others; others – families, care staff – were responsible for *them.* This meant that when they were ill, they could not derive a continued sense of self-worth from such responsibility.

Being the giving partner in relationships with others can give people's life meaning, even during a final illness. Whilst it can be devastatingly difficult to let go of the ability to 'do' things for others, when people are terminally ill they can still give love to their partners, children and friends. Spending time with them becomes more important than anything else. For the people in the Veronica Project, relationships with family members and carers were very important; but most simply didn't have that many significant others in their lives.

Vincent Sweeney's loneliness was painful to witness. He was acutely aware of his unfulfilled need for relationships, his constant longing for family and friends. Many of the men and women in the Veronica Project were deeply lonely. Reciprocal relationships with friends were rare; if people did have friends, they could not sustain such friendships when they were ill. They were utterly dependent on others to support them through life, including organising their relationships and social life.

John Davies gave up his attempts at independence and moved back with his family; he had realised that with the loss of his ability to go out, his life was empty. He had never wanted his friends to visit his flat, but would rather go out to see them; now, he was alone. As has been described earlier, this is his account of life in his flat after surgery for cancer:

> 'The carer would come in and do the housework, and stick me in the bath, the district nurse would come and do the dressing, but if it was raining it got so lonely. I couldn't go anywhere, and if nobody came to visit me, I sat watching the TV or watching the same DVDs over and over again. At one point I could sit there and sing every song from Sister Act I and II with Whoopi Goldberg in. And I would phone people up saying, "Here I am, I'm all right Jack, blah, blah, blah...'

Abandonment and loss

Many of the men and women had a history of being abandoned, starting in early childhood. Dimas, Ursula, Nick, Ben, Richard and Marion had all been removed from their families in childhood to live in institutional settings. Sally also briefly lived in an institution as a toddler. None of the families sent their children away out of malice. However, the effect was that people had suffered terrible losses. The crippling effect of bereavement on people with learning disabilities has only been recognised in recent decades (Blackman 2003; Oswin 1991); before the 1990s people with learning disabilities who suffered a loss were not given any particular consideration. Those in the Veronica Project who had spent their lives in institutions were sometimes described as self-centred, even selfish. It was difficult to get a glimpse of their inner world, as if they had retreated into a world of their own.

Richard thought his mental health problems had started when he was four years old, and he had to be hospitalised for two years because of lung disease. His parents were not allowed to visit. Richard remembered his feelings vividly: 'I know it was because of the infection, but I thought they stopped seeing me because they didn't love me any more.'

Such distress was also described by others who were sent to boarding schools where they were only allowed very limited contact with their families.

People's life stories were stories of loss: the death of beloved parents; being moved away from friends, often without explanation; a succession of paid carers who came and went throughout their lives, carers with whom they had built close bonds. They had no control over such events. Sally Burnett sometimes mentioned her advocate Caroline, whom she liked very much and who had now left. She didn't know where Caroline was, and missed her. Lying in her hospice bed, she sometimes asked people, including myself: 'Where is Caroline?'

Whilst loss is an inevitable part of life for all of us, the profound impact these losses had on the lives of the men and women in the Veronica Project was striking. Parents were deeply mourned, decades after they died. The mention of her father brought immediate tears to Pauline Deweert's eyes, more than 40 years after his death, her memories vivid. It seemed that people had not been given much help during their lives to understand and accommodate their losses.

It is difficult to know the effect of such life histories when people come to face the loss of their own lives. Although they were remarkably resilient, the losses associated with illness and dying were often keenly felt. For Sally Burnett, the loss of mobility was devastating. People's expectations in life were not high, but they cherished their achievements, familiar routines, tasks during the day, loving relatives. 'I'm not ready for heaven yet,' John Davies said nine months before he died. He wanted more songs to sing, more time to spend with his family. Vincent Sweeney wanted to be reconciled with the loss of his father, dreaming of visiting the grave.

Some carers were acutely aware of the hardships people had to endure. After Ursula Smith died, Mary said: 'She looked so peaceful. I was looking at her, and I thought, "You had such a hard life."'

Lack of power and control

Palliative care services aim to focus on the dying person, his needs and wishes. They help the person to make choices. What does he want to do with his remaining time? Where does he want to be cared for, where does he want to die?

Helping people with learning disabilities to make these kind of choices can be challenging. They may not have been allowed to make many decisions in the course of their lives, and therefore have little experience of making real choices. Other people decided for them where they lived, who they lived with, what they did during the day, perhaps even what they ate. The lives of most of the people in the Veronica Project had been heavily supervised, right up to their older years.

People with learning disabilities often have a tendency to agree with those they perceive as more powerful: their families, their support workers, their doctors and nurses. I observed again and again how people said 'yes' even when they may have meant 'no'; how even those who were known for their uncooperative behaviour often meekly followed their carers' demands. 'He won't sit and do his colouring,' one support worker complained about Nick Ballard's refusal to join his elderly fellow residents with their colouring books and pencils – but when she told him to take off his jumper because it was too hot, he complied immediately and without words. I didn't think it was particularly hot, and was wearing a jumper myself.

The people with learning disabilities who managed to 'be in control' relished their freedom. This was why Vincent Sweeney wanted to stay in his flat, despite his loneliness. When I asked Lily Lamb what she liked doing most, she said without hesitation, 'Meetings. Taking decisions.'

Richard Horwood, reflecting on the many places where he had lived (family home, psychiatric hospital, residential care home for people with learning disabilities, and now his own shared flat) had no doubts which he preferred. He said:

> 'I like the house I live in now, best of all. And the worst was the residential home. Why? Now, I can do what I like. I can come and go as I like, and eat whatever I like. In the home, staff treated you like children. They would say things like *[patronising voice]* "Would you like a sweet?", or "Be careful when you cross the road." And they made me wear a bib. I don't have my own teeth so I make a bit of a mess sometimes, but I didn't like having to wear a bib. And you had to finish your food, always, everything that was on your plate.'

When they were ill and dying, other people could exert even more control over their lives. Helena's insistence that Ursula drank her coffee is just one example. Nick Ballard's day centre staff controlled every move he made, employing an extra member of staff to ensure that he didn't go up the stairs, down the stairs, get a cup of coffee before it was coffee time, do some painting when he was supposed to be cooking.

Empty days

Although several people had found activities they enjoyed, maybe even a job, it was hard to escape the conclusion that much of their time was spent simply sitting around. Some day centres didn't always provide meaningful and fulfilling activities, but at least they provided a welcome change. Mary said of the closure of Ursula Smith's day centre ten years ago: 'It killed her.'

The people in the Veronica Project seemed remarkably patient during their illness, and perhaps this was partly because of their long experience of empty days. Sitting around seemed much more difficult for me than for them. Here is a description of a visit to Sally at the hospice:

> *It is hard for me, just sitting here like this. I am used to multitasking; I am tempted to reach for my newspaper, and briefly consider it, as an acceptable way of spending silent time together. But I quickly realise that it would achieve*

the opposite: it would block her out. So I sit, just as she is sitting. And I sit. And I sit…

Another feeling emerges as I am sitting with Sally, and it is the feeling that I am slowly becoming disabled. The tedium of nothing happening, of being so utterly dependent on others to make things happen in your life. Because this boring sitting around is, of course, not new to Sally. Like many people with learning disabilities, she is rather expert at it. She is patient; her expectations of life, of her days, are not high. I can manage it for an hour, but a whole day would probably make me want to scream. Of course, the comparison is slightly unfair, because I am not ill. In her position, physically weak, life very slowly ebbing away, it is not particularly unusual to accept doing absolutely nothing, to preserve energy for visitors. But even so… I think of Nick, people at his home and his day centre, the way their lives were often spent sitting around. We know all these things, but it takes an hour of sitting for me to glimpse just a shimmer of what it feels like.

Not wanting to be a burden

John Davies constantly worried about being a burden to his family:

- 'You don't want to end up in the same position as me, worrying people sick.'
- 'I don't want my mum to take any more trouble.'
- 'I don't want [my family] to see me in terrible pain.'
- 'I'm finding it difficult having people to help me. I find it difficult to say, "Look, I need a push in a wheelchair, because I need to go somewhere"… I'm at the mercy of other people at the minute.'

He wasn't alone in this. Even Vincent Sweeney, who complained a lot, was acutely aware of burdening his family. He said of his sister-in-law:

> 'Susan is always there for me. I can't praise her highly enough. But I can see in her face that it is really too much for her. She has so much on her plate… It shouldn't really be her job to help me.'

Several people with learning disabilities had learnt at an early age to hide their pain and distress. Sometimes this was because of a sense of loss and rejection. For other people it was perhaps because they were already so used to physical pain. Pete Carpenter's deformed feet had caused him to suffer terrible pain in his childhood; now, in the final stages of cancer, he rarely complained. Bob and May explained that Lily Lamb would only complain of pain if it was really bad.

On the one hand, people who had been 'looked after' all their lives expected others to do things for them; but on the other hand, when their support needs increased, they somehow plodded on without asking for extra help.

'Does my life matter?'

Most people in the Veronica Project took an important place within loving, caring families. Yet they also had a lifelong sense of being different, not worthy, less important than other people. This had a far-reaching influence that made itself felt when they were dying. Whilst I was shocked at the way many people were ignored by hospital staff, they themselves did not seem to expect any different.

Being part of the Veronica Project was often helpful to the participants in unexpected ways. To have someone who was interested in their lives, someone who was not a relative or a carer, someone who was there to listen *because their story mattered*...this was hugely empowering to people who were not used to being important. The idea that their stories might be in a book made people's eyes light up with amazed excitement.

This empowering effect was very clear with John Davies, who used the Veronica Project to give meaning to his life and dying. He was both astonished and delighted to find that his story might be of interest to others. Two months after we met, I told his story at a conference, with his consent and active involvement – he had audio-recorded some of his story.

> *The first thing he asks is about the conference. Where exactly was it? I tell him what it was, where it was, and who was there. He wants to know everything, so I describe the huge lecture theatre, and the high-tech IT assistant who played the audio CD bang on cue ('so that was you, your voice, really loud in this big theatre, talking to all these people, and you could hear a pin drop')... I*

tell him that people were very much moved, and some were dabbing their eyes. He is utterly delighted.

'Wow. That's amazing. I can't believe my story had people reaching for their hankies. People said to me, "Who'd want to hear YOUR story?" I know you said you would tell my story, but to be honest I thought it would probably sit at the back of a drawer, and then in some future years people would find it and go, "Oh yeah, here's a story." I didn't really believe anything would really happen with it… That's amazing.'

Despite the many achievements of his life, finding independence, singing in pubs, volunteering with a performing arts company, it was always hard for John to believe, truly, that his life was important, that he mattered. He blossomed during his stay at the hospice, towards the end of his life: 'They treat you like royalty here.' His remark reminded me of something he said many months before, when recounting the death of his friend Paul in a hospice: 'It's an amazing place. They treat you with love and respect.'

Being treated like royalty, with love and respect: a sea-change for the boy who was bullied and who struggled to find his place in the world. Several people sought reassurance from those around them that they deserved a place in the world, and that they were not a burden.

Ben Edwards asked repeatedly, 'Do you like me?' Lily Lamb's nurses came to expect her question: 'Am I a good girl? It's not my fault.' Amanda Cresswell, when recalling how she ran away from an abusive situation, said 'I'm not a naughty person.'

It was as if these men and women tried to convince those around them that they were intrinsically good human beings – and they desperately needed to believe it themselves.

Forced jollity

It is difficult to be with someone in distress. Staying with someone who is deeply unhappy or upset demands commitment and emotional maturity. Bereaved people are often heard to comment that they have discovered who their real friends are: people who have stayed around, who are maybe uncomfortable with the tears, who maybe don't know what to say, but who have nonetheless kept in contact. People who do not cross to the other side of the road to avoid facing them.

However, we would expect most staff in the caring professions to be able to acknowledge sadness in the people they support. I was therefore rather shocked, not only to find how many staff members were in the habit of 'jollying along' a person with learning disabilities who had every reason to be sad, but also to what extent the people with learning disabilities had learned to hide their pain and distress.

Sally Burnett was deeply distressed as she lay in her hospice bed. I wrote in my field notes:

> *During the long silences we spend together, she turns her head to look at me regularly, her mouth curving into a smile that I find difficult to read. Is she happy that I'm here? Or is it simply a learnt smile – one that, she has come to understand, will keep people on her side? I don't know. But it does reassure me. It is not easy to simply sit here, and I need to know that she doesn't mind.*

I discovered that just like the hospice staff, I wanted Sally to smile at me. With each person, it took time before I was able to sit with their distress, and sometimes I never managed it. This is what happened when I sat with Lily Lamb, a week before she died.

> *I sit down next to Lily. I no longer take her hand, because she keeps gesturing with it, and I wonder whether I am actually doing more harm than good, as holding her hand rouses her. Lily remains unsettled. She is beginning to indicate her leg, but I can't make out whether or not she wants it raised on a pillow. She says 'it hurts', and 'pain in leg'. She keeps appealing to me for help that I cannot give; I feel helpless. I keep looking at her face and read the distress in it: the frown, the unhappiness. I am a nurse with many years experience of supporting dying patients, and here I am, sitting next to a woman in her final days, and I cannot bear her distress. I cannot bear sitting here. I want to be the nurse who just came in to help her, who adjusted some pillows, spoke to her gently and warmly, but then left the room again with the promise of more medication if things didn't settle. I want to leave the room too, and go off to do some more wonderful supporting of other dying people in other rooms. I do not want to stay here, and witness Lily's distress.*
>
> *Lily is beginning to ask me to get a nurse, to ring the bell. What can I do? I know the nurses are busy, I know there is probably not much more they can do than I have already tried, yet I also know why Lily wants a nurse. I can feel it. I want a nurse, I want someone to come again and sort us out. As she keeps asking me to ring the bell, I press it. I watch as the magic nurses walk past the door, and I realise more than ever how important it is to be*

acknowledged, as a patient, as a relative. I can hear one of the nurses (whom I know is very busy) say, 'Yes I've heard it [the bell], *but I'm not going to answer it.' After a minute or two – which seems like a long time when you are sitting, waiting, in distress – a nurse walks in. I turn the bell off, I am hugely apologetic, saying what Lily wanted. The nurse does not come into the room completely. She explains to me, in a tone of voice as if she is explaining this to a three-year-old, that the other nurse has just given Lily a painkiller, and that she will give her another one soon. Then she leaves the room, leaving me with a feeling of having done something naughty. I don't really mind, but I do feel just a fraction of the dependence that Lily must be feeling.*

In several of the residential care homes, staff talked to residents in loud and cheery voices, the way people talk to very young children. 'Come on, give us a smile, cheer up!' a support worker urged Ben Edwards when he stared ahead of him with a serious expression. 'We don't want all this grumpiness!' Ben responded by immediately putting on a huge grin. 'That's better,' the support worker said, approvingly.

Nick Ballard's day centre wrote in his care plan that his goal was to 'smile and be happy', and staff frequently encouraged him to smile.

There seemed to be a culture of cheerfulness, even when nobody actually felt cheerful. When people became ill, this façade of jolliness continued. On admission to the hospice, Sally Burnett asked her doctor about her supra-pubic catheter.

'How long do I keep the tube?' Sally asks. The doctor explains, 'The tube was put in your stomach because the water couldn't come out. If we took it out, you would have the same problem again. So it has to stay in. We will teach you how to empty it. You can manage your other bag [colostomy bag], *so you will be able to learn this. We will show you.'*

Joy leans over to her, smiling cheerfully: 'Well, that's good, isn't it! It is easy. It's not as hard as your other bag. You'll be OK.' Sally looks at her, nodding, with her vague reassuring smile, then stares ahead again.

Throughout her hospice stay, Sally was surrounded by staff who encouraged her to sing songs, and who told her that she was doing fine. She wasn't doing fine. She was dying.

It may be that some people respond well to a cheery culture. Sally's stepmother Joy reflected after Sally died that she really did cope well with the supra-pubic catheter, it wasn't a problem for Sally, in fact she found it quite a handy contraption, saving her the effort of having to go to the toilet. However, the hospice staff agreed that Sally often cried. Her physiotherapist said: 'She is all right, quite cheerful, she cries but then she just stops, as if she can't be bothered crying any more.'

I found the sometimes unrelenting jolliness difficult to witness. I wrote in Sally's notes:

> *This may just be my own feelings; but if I were in her shoes, I would want someone to sit down and acknowledge that it is all bloody miserable, it is not going to get any better, and we'll have to make the best of it.*

A desire by staff to keep things jolly was described by Maureen Oswin in her seminal book on bereavement amongst people with learning disabilities. She was one of the first researchers to describe and acknowledge that people with learning disabilities have feelings of sadness and grief.

> One young man, suddenly admitted to a hospital during a weekend because of a parent's death, said, 'They kept wanting me to dance, but I was too sad to.'... There appear to be two standards of expectations regarding emotional reactions to sad experiences, depending on whether a person has a learning difficulty or not: thus, if a person with a learning difficulty agrees to dance following a death his action will be greeted with approval and relief that he is happily occupied; but a person without a learning difficulty going to a dance immediately after a death would be disapproved of. (Oswin 1991, pp.99–100)

Many families and other carers were anxious to keep the person happy. The often-heard statement, 'Why tell him, why upset him, just keep him happy, he is happy as he is' seems to be a continuation of a lifelong desire to keep people with learning disabilities happy. Valerie Sinason, a psychotherapist working with people with learning disabilities who have been abused, noted:

> Guilt that people exist who have to bear unfair and appalling emotional, physical or mental burdens can be so unbearable that a state of denial is brought about where those in greatest pain are asked to be the happiest. (Sinason 1992, p.141)

She noticed that people with learning disabilities responded with what she called 'the handicapped smile': a smile that is not really a smile, but a defence against trauma, hiding profound feelings of pain. Staff, she argued, often collude with this image of happiness.

I found evidence of this kind of collusion, the idea that people with learning disabilities are much happier than the rest of us. This was perhaps most evident at the funerals (see Chapter 8).

Feeling helpless, angry, fearful or guilty is normal when working with people who are dying. It can be difficult for carers to acknowledge the distress and hidden sadness felt by people with learning disabilities, not least because it requires carers to recognise their own distress. Seeing only the good in people and encouraging them to be 'a good girl', to be happy, may well be a defence against carers' own helplessness.

People were good at hiding their pain. Sally Burnett smiled and nodded at her physiotherapist's insistence that things were going well. John Davies explained:

> 'It can be hard. Sometimes I sit in the hospital bed feeling miserable, and I think, "Right, in the next ten minutes they'll all turn up to visit me," so I take a deep breath, put a smile on, and I sit there for half an hour or so talking about silly things. I've done that plenty of times, make out that I'm all right when inside I'm not, I'm just fed up.'

Amanda Cresswell almost whooped with delighted recognition when I read John Davies' words to her. 'Yes! I've done that too!'

'Of course,' agreed Gary Butler, my colleague with learning disabilities who helped me to analyse and think about the Veronica Project. 'We all do that. People with learning disabilities do it all the time.' He was invariably angry about people with learning disabilities not being told difficult truths because 'it might upset them'. 'Why aren't we allowed to be upset?' he asked, but he also knew the answer to his question: 'Because they don't know how to cope with people with learning disabilities being upset.'

The importance of listening

Listening to people's stories was a powerful and important thing to do: not just the story of their illness, but the story of their life. It would have been impossible to consider how people could be best supported when they were dying without taking those life stories into account.

I met many carers who were sensitive, warm, compassionate, loving; carers who understood people's needs and tried hard to meet them. Lily's sister-in-law May was patient and spent many hours every week sitting with Lily, trying to understand what she needed.

Yanna, the home manager, tried hard to understand the meaning of Ben's words and behaviour. She was the only person who realised how unwell he was the day before he died, and called in the family: 'He was just not quite right,' she explained. 'Something was different.' Her careful listening over the years had made her very sensitive to Ben's needs.

Many of the paid staff, families and friends became key figures in people's support at the end of life. Their support took a variety of forms. Vincent's friend Frank, for example, was ready to listen to Vincent at any time of the day or night.

What these key people had in common was a willingness to try to understand the person's life, the importance of his or her relationships and the things that mattered to that person. However, many were also overwhelmed by the burden of care. Life made many demands, and it could be hard to stay focused on the needs of this vulnerable person.

In order to listen more carefully, I found it helpful to focus on the person single-mindedly, and keep these questions in mind:

> 'What matters most to you? For you, having lived this life, having enjoyed and suffered these things, having loved these places and these people; for you, who are now facing this illness, whose life and abilities are now changing so much: how can we support and help you? What is it that matters most *to you*?'

Nobody can answer these questions for anyone else; but people with learning disabilities, who have led such dependent lives, often need others to help them communicate the answers. They need others to listen.

I found that there were several aspects to listening. It was important to be able to 'be' with someone in distress (Tuffrey-Wijne 2009a). This may well be too much for caregivers to bear day after day. I only visited once a week at most; I could go away, reflect, talk to other members of the research team, before going back to listen some more. I wrote after a reflective session with Professor Sheila Hollins:

> *I need help in figuring out how not to run away from it, and how not to crumble under the weight of their pain. This is the trouble with 'truly listening': in trying to understand people's lives from the inside, I have to understand their pain.*
>
> *Sheila compares this to what happens in psychotherapy. How the client puts his emotions into the therapist ('transference'), and the therapist's task is to hold it for him. That is the challenge: simply to hold it, keep it safe, without trying to solve it. One thing I could do is acknowledge the pain, acknowledge how hard it must be, and how important that I know about it.*

Of course daily caregivers cannot, and should not, be asked to act as psychotherapists, but those who are able to acknowledge pain, and to acknowledge that there is nothing they can do, will provide immeasurable support.

Another important aspect of trying to understand 'what matters most' is the ability to let go of any preconceived ideas about what is best for the person. This requires awareness of our own attitudes and opinions, and careful scrutiny of our motivations. For example, we may think that someone should have a rest in the afternoons, but if that person indicates that he would much rather be walking up and down the stairs, does it matter? Why do we insist? Is it truly in the person's best interest? Are the stairs unsafe? Do we lack the resources to ensure he is kept safe? What can we do to meet his needs and wishes?

It was easier for me, as a researcher, to let go of my own needs and wishes. I did not have any formal 'helping' role, and I did not need to support the people in the Veronica Project. The value of my listening role was put into words by Vincent Sweeney. When I told him that it was not my job to help him, but simply to listen to him and to try to understand him, he said, 'That's good enough for me. It really helps me, talking to you. Unburdening myself.'

I was probably the only person to whom Vincent confessed that he threw most of his medication in the bin. Although the district nurses neatly arranged them in a weekly box, he found it hard to understand the proliferation of tablets, and preferred to take only the ones he knew were for pain. He needed to feel that he was in control of his tablets. Vincent told me this during a long conversation about his cancer worries and his loneliness. I knew that his hospice nurse was at her wits' end trying to find an effective medication regime, and his family were desperate for him to comply with the doctors. It suddenly became clear why Vincent had told me but not anyone else: I was the only person unlikely to try to tell him what to do, and the only person unlikely to tell anyone else what he'd said.[11] When his sister-in-law asked him a question, she knew what answer she wanted to hear; if Vincent's answer didn't measure up, she gave him that 'right' answer almost before he had finished speaking. She had her own agenda. It occurred to me that if I was his palliative care nurse, I too would have my agenda. I would listen, yes, but I would have the 'What can I give him for his pain?' question prominently in my mind. I would probably focus mostly on the physical effects of his cancer, and how they could be dealt with. It would hinder my listening.

(Later, when Susan had read this paragraph in preparation for publishing this book, she rang me and said: 'You were right, you know, about him not taking his medication. After he died, we found whole stacks of them that he'd hidden away in his kitchen cupboard. We suspected it, but we never knew for sure. He always said he took them.')

Finally, answering the question 'What matters most to you?' may simply be a matter of listening to what someone has been trying to say all along. Most people told me about the important aspects of their lives in my very first meeting with them, but sometimes I was too focused on the questions in my own mind to appreciate the significance of their words and actions.

Ben Edwards had very little speech, and the few words he said were hard to understand. When I first met him at his residential care home, he repeated the names of his brother and sister-in-law until, with the help of his support worker, I managed to understand what he said. He then dragged me upstairs and proudly showed me his room: his own bed and television, the posters of Cliff Richard, the videos stacked high in every corner. He frowned as he mimed how people had hit him in the past. He mentioned various outings during the week.

I met Ben towards the end of the Veronica Project, and I had learnt not to come with any clear ideas about what I needed to focus on, even during a first visit. Yet what I learnt about him during those first few hours did not change over the course of the year. He had shown me that his family were tremendously important to him. He liked having his own space, with his music and videos. He didn't want to sit at home all day; he liked going out; he didn't like people being cruel or rough. These issues were important for his future care. His family needed to be involved as much as possible. Where should he be cared for when he became weaker – could he stay at home? If not, where else would he feel safe and in control? Where else could he have a space of his own, with his television and videos? The importance of his outings and activities had to be remembered. And throughout all this, Ben wanted carers to be considerate and kind.

Ben's carers were aware of his needs and wishes. They worked hard at keeping him at home until he died, and at helping him to have contact with his family. A few weeks before he died, they encouraged him to join his family for his mother's ninetieth birthday party, even though his relatives were doubtful. They weren't sure Ben was well enough. It turned out to be hugely important, giving Ben much joy that sustained him, and giving his family some precious memories. Ben's sister had come over for the party from America, and this was their final chance to see each other.

Summary

- It was very important to understand people's life stories. Their experience of life affected their experience of cancer and dying.
- All 13 people communicated what was important to them, but it needed sensitivity to appreciate the significance of their

words and actions. It was important to listen, and to try to understand what mattered most to them.

- People with learning disabilities were dependent on others throughout their lives.
- They had all experienced bullying and abuse, including verbal, physical, financial and sexual abuse.
- When they were ill and dying, they were even more vulnerable to abuse of power. I witnessed one incident of institutional abuse of a terminally ill woman with severe learning disabilities by a support worker.
- People with learning disabilities were not perceived as adults with a sexual identity.
- Only one person had an acknowledged partner, and none had children. For some people, the lack of a partner caused a deep sense of loss at the end of life.
- Many people were very lonely. When they were ill, they could not maintain friendships without help.
- People with learning disabilities had a lifelong history of loss and abandonment, through bereavements and moves into residential care. Several people were still mourning early losses.
- People with learning disabilities lacked power and control over their lives. Others made decisions for them in many areas of living. Some had very limited experience of making choices, and were used to being told what to do. Those who had achieved a degree of independence, or were encouraged to be involved in making decisions, valued this very highly.
- Many people with learning disabilities were remarkably patient. They were used to the fact that not much happened in their daily lives.
- Several people worried about being a burden to their families.

- There was a sense among the people with learning disabilities that their lives were unimportant. Some, including people with severe learning disabilities, sought repeated reassurance that others liked them.
- There was a strong tendency among staff to 'jolly along' people with learning disabilities, even if that person had good reason to be sad. Several learning disability services had a culture of 'jolliness', frequently encouraging residents to smile and be cheerful. Some families and health care staff also kept up a cheerful façade.
- People with learning disabilities were good at hiding their pain and distress; they often pretended that everything was well.
- It could be very difficult, and sometimes unbearable, to stay with someone in distress and acknowledge his or her feelings; yet this was what people needed. It may not be possible, or necessary, to 'do' anything; sometimes the most powerful thing others could do for them was to 'be with' them.
- There were many sensitive, loving carers who tried hard to listen and understand the person with learning disabilities.

CHAPTER 7

Resilience

'Don't let life get to you. Don't let cancer get to you.' This is how my colleague Gary Butler, who has learning disabilities himself, summed up the theme that had struck him all the way through reading people's stories. It is the reason why, despite all the misery, he felt inspired and uplifted by these stories.

It is easy to focus on the limitations of people with learning disabilities, on the things they cannot do and the support they need, on the hardships of their lives. We may well expect them to have difficulties in coping with the uncertainties, changes and losses associated with cancer and death. Many, as we have seen, did find it hard. But that is not the full story. There were also unexpected triumphs and resilience in the face of adversity. I often left people with a smile on my face.

This chapter looks at resilience in people with learning disabilities who have cancer and who are dying. I will look closely at how people coped with deteriorating health and approaching death. What kept them going?

The story of Richard Horwood illustrates resilience very well.

Richard Horwood: 'Don't ever give up'

Richard Horwood was 64 years old and had mild learning disabilities. I was introduced to him by the staff at a day centre for people with learning disabilities, which he had attended for the past 20 years, dropping in for a few hours once or twice a week. He enjoyed the activities there, and dipped in and out of them as he pleased.

Richard lived semi-independently in a small house he shared with his friend Charlie. They had moved in together seven years ago from a residential care home for people with learning disabilities. Richard had a caring group of professionals around him: a dedicated case manager from social services; a key worker; his learning disability nurse; someone who accompanied him to all his medical appointments; a team of support workers. He received 30 hours of support per week, for shopping, cooking, cleaning and managing his finances. He didn't like strangers in the house and would usually refuse any suggestion of a new support worker or extra help, until he had met the person: 'Oh, if it's him, it's all right.' His flat was usually strewn with papers and other bits and pieces. His flat mate Charlie was a competent, no-nonsense type of person, answering the telephone, relaying messages, and helping the support workers by telling them exactly what had happened and who had already been in contact. He had a busy social life with friends and clubs. Richard also took part in some of Charlie's activities, but most of the time he just liked to go for walks, roaming about town. His house was a 20-minute bus ride from the town centre. He loved to catch the bus, have a wander, find himself some lunch in a café, maybe drop into the day centre, and come home in his own good time. After a lifetime in care, he relished the independence.

Richard was a tall and slightly stooped man. He walked a little unsteadily, leaning on his walking stick. His appearance could be off-putting, with food remnants stuck in the unshaven corners of his mouth, sometimes surrounded by a faint smell of unwashed clothes and stale urine; but he had friendly eyes and generous smile. Those who knew him described him as a 'gentle giant'. Once, talking about the drama group he attended, I asked him what role he would choose for himself, if he could be anything he liked. Would he play a goodie or a baddie? He looked at me, laughing out loud. 'A goodie! I couldn't be a baddie. I wouldn't know how to be a baddie. It's not in my nature.'

Richard didn't like talking about the difficult things that had happened in his younger years, but they still haunted him. He had battled with depression all his life. Here is one conversation I had with him, seven months after we met.

'We could talk some more about all that,' I suggest. 'The good times and the bad times.' 'I've had quite a few bad times,' he says immediately. I don't really

leave a long enough silence before asking him about the bad times – silences with Richard often seem rather uncomfortable for some reason. 'Do you want to tell me about those?' 'Not really,' he says, and it is as if the shutters have gone down. He was open and cheerful so far, but now he is staring at the ground, not looking at me, sadly pensive. 'That's OK,' I say. 'It can be too difficult sometimes, thinking about the bad times.' This time I do leave a little silence, and he fills it by saying, 'I don't want to talk about that.'

'How about the good times, then?' I ask. 'They are important too.' He looks up immediately, his eyes twinkling. 'Oh yes!'

Staff at the day centre placed a strong emphasis on happiness, often trying to make him smile or urging him to tell one of his jokes.

Growing up

Richard was the second of four children. Apart from a two-year spell in hospital in early childhood, Richard lived with his family. It was a loving family, maintaining strong bonds that lasted into adulthood. He spoke warmly of his parents, the way they would never hit him if he had been naughty, but rather punish him by taking away certain privileges, like forbidding him to go out walking for a week. That was punishment indeed. He loved walking, even at a young age.

'I was in the newspaper once, because my mother had phoned the police! I was 14 years old. My picture in the newspaper! She had given me up as a missing person. I had gone for a long walk, all the way from London to Oxford. I had heard about a man who had walked that far, and I thought: "I'm a man, if he can do it, I can." So I wanted to try. I did tell my mother where I was going, but she was still worried and she called the police because she couldn't find me. I was gone for a week, because it took me a week to get there. Then when I got to Oxford, the police picked me up. My mother had given a description of what I looked like. Then my father came to collect me in his 1958 car and drove me home.'

He is aware of how deliciously unusual his escapade is, and he loves the effect on me of telling this story. He doesn't seem to see it as naughty or stupid: didn't he tell his mother where he was going? Why shouldn't a boy of 14 want to go off for a long walk? 'Where on earth did you sleep?' I want to know. 'Oh, just in bus shelters,' he explains, as if it is the most obvious thing in the world. And no, his mother was not angry when he came back. I suggest that she was probably just relieved to have him back, and he agrees.

Despite these happy memories, Richard's childhood was not always easy. His mother was a sensitive person who suffered from depression; his maternal grandfather had also struggled with mental illness. Richard thought that he had inherited these tendencies. The separation from his family when he had to be hospitalised was painful. He was bullied at school and continued to be bullied as an adult.

Richard was admitted to a psychiatric hospital when he was 18, and stayed there for eight years before going back home to live with his parents again. He had many unhappy memories of the institution.

> 'I saw things in that hospital that you wouldn't see today, like staff beating patients. I was never beaten myself, but I saw staff beating other patients every day, four times a day. And I couldn't do anything about it, because if I said anything, the staff would say, "He is imagining things." You can't do anything when you are a patient. That was terrible.'

When he was in his late forties, Richard moved into a residential home for people with learning disabilities (where he met Charlie). He helped the less able residents with simple tasks, like making the tea, but learnt some new skills himself too. His mother had done everything for him, and he wasn't used to looking after himself. But when the opportunity came to move into his current house and be more independent, he took it with both hands; he hated the residential care home even more than he had hated the psychiatric hospital. He hated being dependent, being treated like a child.

Cancer

Richard's family were deeply shocked but not surprised by his diagnosis of lung cancer. He was a steady smoker with a history of heart problems, and the cancer was picked up during a bronchoscopy as part of the investigations related to his heart. It is unclear whether Richard had any signs or symptoms of cancer beforehand; if he had pain or had felt unwell, he certainly hadn't told anyone.

He was offered a course of four radiotherapy treatments, but only received one. He thought radiotherapy was 'like an X-ray', but didn't quite understand what it was meant to do. I was told by his support workers that the cancer was 'terminal', but nobody quite knew whether Richard understood this. Richard was always very clear that he had cancer in his lung, and that this was the cause of his increasing tiredness and pain, although it only dawned on him gradually, as his health deteriorated over the course of the next two years, that he would not survive the cancer. He dealt with this knowledge in a matter-of-fact way.

Richard carried tablets in his pocket to help with the pain, but they didn't take the pain away completely. He was rather resigned to this, as if pain was an inevitable part of cancer. Things improved when, months later, he started taking morphine tablets. If he had the slightest health complaints – and this happened quite regularly – Richard took himself to the Accident and Emergency department at the nearby hospital, rather than to his GP. He knew how to get there, and he knew the staff would help him. The Accident and Emergency staff had indeed learnt how to 'deal with him'.

Coping with the loss of independence

The main effect of cancer on Richard's life was his increasing weakness and tiredness, affecting his ability to walk. Support workers held their breath as he continued to wander about town, unsteady on his feet, even more vulnerable than he had already been. But there was no question of him stopping these walks, these expressions of his freedom. Once, when I asked him what life would be like if he couldn't walk any more, he answered even before I had finished speaking: 'Oh, that would be terrible.'

He needed more support at home, and he gradually relented, agreeing to increased help with the housekeeping (he could no longer carry his own washing down the stairs) and, eventually, help with washing and dressing. After protracted negotiations, a stair lift was put in, as it had become almost impossible for him to negotiate the stairs up to his bedroom.

As the months progressed, he needed to spend more time resting, often coming home after only a short time in town. Sometimes he didn't get up until 3pm. The professionals and the family were genuinely concerned about what would happen to him when he was no longer able to manage in his house. Already, Charlie felt under pressure. Richard was worried about falling and often asked Charlie to stay at home. Richard had fallen once and he didn't want to be on his own. The professionals acknowledged that Richard's hard-won independence was the single most important thing for him. He was usually very polite about any suggestions of how to manage, but then simply disregarded them. He would not take kindly to any loss of his ability to do as he liked. His case manager said fondly, 'He is the most lovable, wonderful, difficult bugger I know.'

To everyone's surprise, it was Richard himself who suggested that he should not live in his own flat any more. Two years after our first meeting, he told me about his decision to move into a nursing home.

> *I remind him: 'In the past, you have said that your flat was the best place you had ever lived. You really didn't like the idea of ever having to go into a home again. Has that now changed?'*
>
> *'Well, I can't be in my own flat,' he says simply. 'So the nursing home is better. I wouldn't want to go back to my own house, because I would worry what happens when I am weak. Who is going to look after me? I have to be realistic. I can't wash myself. I can wash my top half, but I can't do the bottom half. It hurts when I bend over. I think that's what cancer does to you. And I am wearing a pad now, because I kept having accidents. That's because of the pills I take. Pills for pain and for cancer, they make you go to the toilet. Sometimes I have to go three times in the night. So it is much better like this, I am well cared for. I feel comfortable and safe in the nursing home.'*
>
> *'You have to be realistic,' he continues. 'I don't dwell on things. I get really annoyed when people get angry. I never get angry. What's the point? I like to think about good things.'*
>
> *'Do you ever lie awake at night, or worry about what might happen to you?' I ask him. 'No, never', he says, and I believe him. He has looked cheerful throughout our conversation, looking at me regularly with a broad grin, and this time I don't sense that it is the smile of someone trying to hide painful feelings. In the past, I have sometimes felt heavy and downcast when I spent time with him. Today, I feel uplifted, and I think that reflects his own mood, a state of being that is genuinely content. I am amazed at his resilience.*

Richard enjoyed the fact that he could simply ring the bell and ask for a cup of tea; the nurses would bring him one, even if it was his third cup in the middle of the night. He preserved his energies for the things he enjoyed. He did as he pleased. He now used a walking frame, and was often found outside, smoking. He still went out for walks. 'We couldn't stop him, even if we wanted to,' one of his nurses said.

Having followed Richard for two years, I told him that I thought he was amazing. 'You have cancer, you have had all these things happening to you, getting weaker...and you just keep going! Look at you, you are still getting out and about!' Richard thought about this, then smiled at me. 'Yeah, I suppose I *am* quite amazing. I don't give up. Don't ever give up. Whatever happens.'

The features of resilience

What is it that makes some people cope with difficult and adverse situations, bounce back from them even, whilst others don't? What makes some people resilient? Half a century ago, researchers became interested in resilience when they noticed that some children from disadvantaged backgrounds survived and even thrived, whilst others could not escape a lifetime of misery. More recently, professionals in palliative care have also started to wonder what makes some people resilient, and 'regularly testify to the many examples of ordinary people achieving extraordinary things in the face of impending loss' (Monroe and Oliviere 2007, p.1).

Not everyone in the Veronica Project found it easy to keep going when they were ill. Ursula Smith struggled with mental health problems. Vincent was an angry man, ready to lash out in order to protect himself. But the majority showed remarkable resilience in the face of ill health and declining abilities.

This was only a small group of people, and I can't claim to have found that 'people with learning disabilities are resilient'. It is, nevertheless, worth looking at the features of resilience among these men and women, and learning from it so that we can try to promote resilience in others by harnessing their strengths.

Experienced sufferers

When I first met Amanda Cresswell, I said that she could tell me as little or as much as she liked, and that I was interested in everything – not only the story of her cancer, but also the story of her life. She agreed immediately that her life story was important: 'Because I think it started as soon as I was born. That's when I had to start fighting.' Amanda went on to describe how she suffered brain damage at birth, and how the hospital priest was called in for a quick christening. She smiled broadly: 'Because I was so small, they really didn't think I would survive. But I proved everybody wrong! I *did* survive!'

People did survive, they survived difficult births and childhoods full of bullying and loneliness. Out of necessity, they found strengths within themselves to cope with the things life had thrown at them. John Davies said: 'I've learned to think, "sticks and stones break my bones"...and I just kept plodding along, going along in my own little way doing this and that.'

The difficulties people had faced in coping with their disability gave them a lifelong training in coping with adversity. They benefited from this experience when they became ill. Cancer, it seemed, was just one more misfortune in a long life of hardship. Families and other carers resented the unfairness of this, but the people themselves often just took it in their stride.

I sometimes wondered whether many people with learning disabilities were actually better prepared for the hardships of terminal illness than most of us. There was a certain amount of self-selection among the participants in the Veronica Project, possibly favouring those who were more resilient. John and Amanda probably took part precisely because they were more flexible, they wanted and were able to give, they had learned to turn their disadvantages into an advantage.

Living in the present moment

People with cancer, whether they have learning disabilities or not, need to find ways of living with the knowledge that life may change in a way that is unimaginable and devastating. One way of coping is to learn to 'take each day as it comes'. As I said earlier, it is not unusual to hear a cancer patient say, 'I am living much more in the moment now. I try to enjoy every day, because you never know what will happen next.'

'Living in the moment' is a skill that many people with learning disabilities already possess. This may be largely due to their cognitive limitations. The ability to worry about the future requires a sense of time and the ability to think in abstract concepts. Not surprisingly, those with more severe learning disabilities were most able to 'live in the moment'. Ben Edwards sat cheerfully in the hospital waiting room, the only patient who did not seem worried about what the doctor was going to say. People who could not understand the meaning and impact of cancer were protected from worrying about it.

But it wasn't just those with severe learning disabilities who seemed to accept matter-of-factly the changes a new day could bring. Several people who had good verbal ability used the word 'realistic'. Richard was 'realistic' when his weakening body forced him to think about nursing homes. When John Davies' mother was suddenly taken into hospital, and his family was trying to reassure him that all would be well, he knew otherwise. John said:

> 'I know I have to be realistic. She may not come home. And if she does come home, she cannot look after me. And I can't look after myself. So I will need to find somewhere else to live. I am very ill, and she can't look after me.'

Both these men were fiercely independent, but they showed a strong sense that it was no use crying over spilt milk. No need to make things seem better than they are: just acknowledge the situation, and get on with it.

Many people in the Veronica Project seemed to have the ability to assess their present situation, come up with a realistic solution to the problem facing them, and then carry it through. They understood the need to move into other care settings when they were ill. Lily Lamb did not think about the possible advantages and joys of being at home in her own surroundings: 'I have pain, I should be in hospital.' Marion Prentice was quite happy to have the 'bad breast' taken off; in the words of her support worker, 'She did not want a messy breast,' and having a mastectomy clearly made sense to her. Sally Burnett coped well with her new urinary catheter. She knew that there was a blockage and she couldn't pass urine herself any more, so the bag was a handy solution.

Not everyone coped equally well. Some were unhappy about their admission to hospital or hospice, missing the securities of home. Sally Burnett cried with longing for her flat. The problem for her was that her carers had set her the unrealistic goal to try to get stronger, causing her much distress. Sally was much better able to cope with the realistic short-term goals of a short visit to her flat: she got ready with much anticipation, getting up early, washing her hair, waiting in her wheelchair for the taxi to arrive.

Experience of being cared for

For people in the general population, loss of independence is often a terribly difficult aspect of terminal illness. Many dying people are more afraid of losing control than they are of physical pain. The loss of hard-won independence could be devastating for people with learning disabilities; yet there was also a clear advantage in having lived dependent lives. Accepting help with the tasks of daily living was not new for them; most were already highly dependent on others.

Their experience of 'having things done for them' extended to being experienced in 'having decisions taken for them'. People's lives could be severely limited by a lack of power; but when it came to terminal illness, the loss of power and control many of us would rail against was nothing new for the people in the Veronica Project. They seemed resigned to it.

Many people with learning disabilities have multiple health problems. Most people in the Veronica Project had experience of hospitals, having endured numerous hospitalisations during their lives. This experience was an advantage when they had cancer. Not everyone liked hospitals, doctors, nurses and needles; but at least they understood what hospitals were all about, and some were experienced patients, offering their arm willingly for blood tests and lifting their shirt for X-rays.

Being 'a cancer patient', not 'someone with learning disabilities'

Vincent Sweeney loved the hospice day centre, mostly because of the contact with other cancer patients. Here, he was not defined by his learning disabilities, not by his mental health problems or alcoholism, but by cancer, something that can happen to absolutely anyone.

The people in the Veronica Project had no problems fitting in with life in a nursing home, hospice ward or day centre: they had experience of being in institutions. They were used to receiving help. In this respect they were unlike many patients without learning disabilities.

Having cancer seemed to make people with learning disabilities more equal to others. They were no longer the only people who had clear limitations.

Like Vincent, Lily Lamb loved the hospice day centre. In the outside world, she was insecure and self-conscious; but here, she was one of many people who had limitations. The following describes her interaction with a fellow patient. He was new to the day centre, and he was nervous. Whilst the other patients were chatting and busying themselves with craft work, he and Lily sat next to each other in silence.

> *He is becoming more relaxed, and is beginning to smile and interact with the other patients. He then takes Lily's hand, looks at her, and says, sounding concerned, 'Are you OK?' She looks back at him with her big observing eyes, and says she is OK. He holds her hand for a few seconds, but she then folds her own hands so he lets go. A little while later, I see him holding her hand again.*
>
> *I am quite touched by this gesture – it is not at all condescending, but more a gesture of support, a recognition of being in the same boat. I am not sure whether the other patients even realise that Lily has learning disabilities. I expect they simply think she is rather ill, with her tired-looking face, her half-open mouth and protruding bottom lip, the frequent dropping of her head on her chest with half-shut eyes before she looks up again to watch what is going on. Many hospice patients lose alertness and ability to speak clearly, maybe due to fatigue, strokes or brain tumours… When I take Lily away, I say 'Bye everyone', and there is a friendly chorus from the patients of 'Goodbye!' The nice thing is that this is not directed at me, but at Lily. She gives them a little wave.*

Having someone who cares

The presence of one or two trusted carers made a huge difference to people's ability to cope. This could be a family member or a support worker. What mattered was that there was someone who knew the person intimately, who was present throughout the illness, and who had formed a deep emotional bond.

It is difficult to imagine how Lily Lamb would have coped without Bob and May. Nick Ballard found life much easier when his home manager Mary was around. Ben Edwards needed his family, but whenever he was upset he called for his home manager Yanna, and she was deeply committed to him, coming in on days off, in the middle of the night if necessary. Vincent Sweeney and John Davies were very clear that their families kept them going. Sally Burnett loved her stepmother, and needed her.

These are not just the stories of the people with learning disabilities; they are also the stories of those who loved and supported them. Without such support, it was much more difficult to cope. These carers were a safety net; people looked out for them at all times. Lily Lamb wanted to know exactly on what day and at what time Bob would return. Nick Ballard wanted Mary to stay with him.

What seemed to help people was the deep knowledge that there was someone who had their best interest at heart; someone who cared. What they needed, more than anything else, was *someone who loved them.* The presence of a key person who could give love was important in bringing out people's resilience. As Dame Cicely Saunders said, 'Suffering is only intolerable if nobody cares' (Saunders 1960).

Keep on going…

There was one aspect of people's coping that was striking to everyone involved. The people with learning disabilities had developed trusted routines; there were activities they loved; and they wanted to keep these going. 'He is amazing, he just keeps going,' families and carers told me over and over again, often with a sense of wonder and admiration.

Richard Horwood kept walking, to the exasperation of his carers who thought he was getting far too weak. John Davies tried to ignore his weakness and pain, focusing instead on the songs he wanted to keep singing, grabbing the microphone at karaoke night and recording a DVD when he was close to death. Others wanted to carry on going to their day centre, even when they were clearly too ill to participate. 'Work in the morning, boys, go to work!' Pete Carpenter said on the day before he died. He carried on rolling cigarettes even when he could hardly smoke them.

People relied on such familiar activities and routines. They were distressed when structure and security were taken away. Vincent Sweeney could not cope when he was no longer able to go to work;

he didn't know how to fill his days. The hospice day centre fulfilled some of his need for structure and human contact, and took his mind off his worries, but it wasn't enough. The four walls of his flat were closing in on him. He explained:

> 'I sit on the sofa, and I just stare at that bit of carpet over there, and thoughts go round and round in my head, and I'm frightened. I am not coping on my own. I need people around me.'

Cancer and dying brings huge uncertainty, and a loss of familiar routines and activities is inevitable. This is hard for most people, not just those with learning disabilities. However, people with learning disabilities are often more reliant than others on the structure of their day. The activities they enjoy may well be more limited. Many people with learning disabilities do not understand why routines need to change, or simply do not have alternatives to fill their lives with. Changes of routine can be particularly distressing for people with a disorder on the autism spectrum, who often prefer their life to be predictable.

It may be unsurprising, therefore, that most people fiercely resisted any changes in routines. They held on, with dogged determination, to the things they enjoyed. The support they received in 'keeping going' was often crucial in how well they coped. Some, like Richard, kept going regardless of what people said ('We can't stop him'), but others relied on their carers to support their wishes. Pete Carpenter was taken to his day centre despite his inability to participate.

Some carers were able to be flexible, even when the person was so frail that his or her choice did not seem sensible. These carers' ability to accommodate the person's wishes could prevent unnecessary distress. Mary said, a few weeks before Ursula Smith died:

> 'She likes sitting in her armchair. Sometimes when she is tired I try to see if she can be in bed, but she doesn't like it. Bed is for night time. The other day she was having a sore bottom from sitting, so I helped her to lie on her side in her bed, but she didn't like it. After an hour she was screaming. She likes to stick to her routine, she likes things to be the same every time. She just keeps going.'

Summary

Most people with learning disabilities were remarkably resilient in the face of declining health. The following aspects helped them to cope with their illness:

- They were 'experienced sufferers' with a lifelong training in coping with adversity. Cancer seemed just one more misfortune in a long life of hardship.
- They were skilled at 'taking each day as it comes'. Those with more severe learning disabilities were particularly good at living in the present moment.
- People with learning disabilities were realistic about their immediate future; for example, they understood the need to go into a nursing home when they were unable to look after themselves. Most people coped best with realistic short-term goals.
- Terminal illness often means a loss of independence. All the people with learning disabilities, including those who had gained a degree of independence, already had extensive experience of being helped and cared for.
- Being a cancer patient meant that people were identified as part of a group of 'people with cancer' that consisted of people in the general population, rather than just as 'people with learning disabilities'. This could be empowering for some.
- The presence of one or two trusted, loving carers or relatives was important in harnessing people's resilience.
- People with learning disabilities wanted to 'keep going' with routines and familiar activities, right up to their final days. They coped best if they were enabled to hold on to their routines and activities.

CHAPTER 8

Dying and Beyond

John, Vincent, Nick, Lily, Pete, Sally, Dimas, Marion, Ben and Ursula had died by the time I finished writing this book. Richard lived with terminal illness; only Amanda and Pauline had been able to pick up their lives, one hopes free of cancer.

The death of someone you have known is always extraordinary. Time stands still – and when time starts to move once more, life can never be the same again. The death of someone we knew and loved brings in its wake feelings of disbelief and distress. How could this happen? We feel shaky, numb, insecure. Death confronts us with issues of love and loss, and brings home to us the fragility of life.

The close bonds formed by families and friends, as well as by many paid carers who supported the people in the Veronica Project on a daily basis, meant that their deaths had a profound impact on them. They had seen the weakness and the deterioration; they may have been told that someone was close to death; yet when the person died, they were deeply shaken. People were rarely prepared for death.

Perhaps the deaths of these men and women were no different from the deaths of people in the general population. Some deaths were slow; others were sudden and unexpected, despite the cancer. These processes of dying seemed unaffected by the presence of learning disability; but they are worth telling. Having followed people's stories, we want to know what happened to them in the end.

After people's deaths and funerals, I kept in touch with many of the carers and families, sometimes for years afterwards. People's stories would not be complete without looking at how their loved ones fared without them.

Lily Lamb's death

When Lily's condition deteriorated, the hospice staff told her family that she could stay. Lily became bed-bound and gradually more sleepy in her final weeks, but she was never completely settled. She remained restless at times. Twelve days before she died, she asked Bob a couple of seemingly important questions. 'Am I going to stay here now?' Bob confirmed that she was. Lily responded that this (the hospice) was her new home then. Later that day, she became more and more distressed, frequently calling out and crying, talking of pain. Lily also expressed her distress at her situation, getting more muddled, often not remembering things, often asking the same question twice, something she had never done before. 'What is happening to me? Why can't I remember things?' She was distressed about her pain, saying repeatedly that 'it's not my fault'.

Lily died early one morning, without any particular warning; there had been no change overnight. The ward sister explained, 'When the night sister popped into her room before she went off duty, she literally took her last breath.'

Lily's funeral was attended by around 45 people: family (mainly May's, as Lily and Bob did not have many relatives left), past and present carers, the people Lily shared her home with. There were also two hospice nurses. One nurse said that attending funerals was rather frowned upon by her superiors. In her job, you could be attending several funerals a week. 'But you know, I just had to come. I was really really fond of Lily. We all were.'

Afterwards, everyone gathered at Lily's home, congregating around large platters of food that May had organised. It was an opportunity to talk to each other and remember Lily. People commented on how much she would have approved of the party, although, May pointed out with fond laughter, not of the plate of fruit. She never liked fruit.

The years that followed were not easy for Bob and May. May's father needed a lot of care; he came to live with them, and died a year after Lily. Her sister also needed support. Bob fell and broke his leg, and eventually retired from his job. Two years later I asked Bob in what way he missed Lily. His eyes immediately filled with tears.

'Oh yes… I do miss her. I don't think of her all the time, but not a week goes by that I am not reminded of her. Something happens and

I think of her, the way she was, the things she said and did. I know she was different maybe, but you know, she was my sister, she was just Lily. I miss the funny things she said sometimes, the laughs we had together…' He trailed off. 'Yes, I do miss Lily and my dad.'

'We have a little graveyard near here,' May continued for him, 'and that's where his mum and dad are, and Lily's ashes are there too. We go there sometimes… I don't think it's sunk in yet. Not fully. That she is not here any more.'

'I think she will always be there,' said Bob. 'It will never go away. She will always be part of us.'

Dying

Pauline Deweert's father died four decades ago, yet she still remembered it clearly: 'It was a rainy day.'

People often have vivid memories of their loved one's last days and hours. They mull over them again and again, trying to make sense of them, trying to read meaning into them, trying to understand. They ask themselves whether they could, or should, have done things differently.

Families and carers told me on the phone what had happened during the days before someone died, at the moment of death, and immediately afterwards. They repeated the story when I saw them. They came back to it during the following months. They told me because I asked them about it; but without exception, people were only too glad to tell me, and tell me again.

Several carers had feelings of uncertainty, even guilt about what had happened. Mary asked, months after Nick Ballard's death: 'Did we do the right thing? Did we do everything that was possible?' The thought that he shouldn't have rung the ambulance when Pete died tormented Ramesh for months afterwards.

Such persisting feelings of guilt about what was done or what was not done could be agonising. People went back over the person's life and illness, trying to find points in history where the course of life and death might have been changed. Maybe if we had noticed his symptoms sooner… What if I had taken her home from hospital?… If only…

Such thoughts and emotions are a normal part of grieving, but I found that few people were prepared for them. Paid carers, in particular, were taken aback by the strength of their emotions. It wasn't part of their job description.

The process of dying

Many cancer patients spend their last days or hours in a state of reduced consciousness, when it is clear to the people around them that they are dying. This gives their loved ones the opportunity to sit with them and to say goodbye. Death, when it comes, is still a shock; it is still hard; but carers can derive comfort from the knowledge that they were there for at least some of the time. It can be an important and intense time, when people are drawn in and focused on the life and death of this one person. Nothing else matters.

Being able to spend the last days and hours with a beloved person was comforting. Mary and her family were gently present when Nick was dying, Mary's eight-year-old daughter resting her head on his stomach. Sally Burnett died with her family at her bedside. My notes describe what happened:

> *Sally died in the hospice early on Saturday morning. Her stepmother Joy and her brother Nigel both stayed the night with her; her sister Vera visited the day before. Joy told me what had happened.*
>
> *On Friday, Sally called out a few times: 'Mum! Mum!' Joy answered: 'I'm here, love. What's up? We're all here. Nigel is here and Vera is here.'*
>
> *'Then she did a funny thing,' Joy continues. 'She was restless, and then suddenly she clapped her hands three times. Now why would she do that? Was she remembering how we used to clap? Or did she see someone?' 'Who knows...' I respond. 'It's such a mystery, isn't it?' 'You're telling me!' says Joy.*
>
> *During the night, Nigel and Joy took it in turns to lie down and rest for a few hours. At 4.45am, Nigel woke his stepmother to say that Sally's breathing had changed. It became more shallow. At 6.40am, her breathing stopped.*
>
> *'I thought: that's it,' says Joy. 'But then after a while it started again. That happened three times. After the third time, I whispered to her, "Time to go, darling." Then, the fourth time, it didn't start again. It was ten minutes to seven.'*

Some people died so quickly that carers were unprepared. There may have been a marked deterioration (Pete Carpenter had not got out of bed; Ursula Smith was drowsy) but no one was aware that death was imminent. This could be difficult, particularly if carers were not able to be present. Mary telephoned me in the early evening to explain how she had left Ursula in hospital, and how unwell Ursula had been.

> 'I left her for about an hour, and when I came back she said, "Are you going to take me home?" So I said to her, "You can't go home yet, you are not well at the moment." She was a bit sad. But then she started to be a bit drowsy, and so I left her in the afternoon... You know, yesterday, when I saw all this, how hard it was for her in hospital, I had tears in my eyes. I said to the doctors, "She is so dear to me. I'd rather take her home." If they're not doing anything, even if they would say that she is dying, that she only has a couple of days, I would take her home. I'd make her comfortable. I'd much rather do that, than have her in hospital. Like we did with Nick. You know?'

A few hours later, Mary telephoned me again, deeply distressed. The nurses had just rung her: Ursula had died. The following day, she filled in the details.

> 'In the evening, she asked the nurses for tea at about 9 o'clock. I don't know how long she had to wait for the tea, but they said that when they came back with the tea, she had died... I went to see her last night.'

Later, I read in Ursula's notes the simple last sentence: 'Went to the hospital to say goodbye.'

The deaths of John Davies and Vincent Sweeney were particularly distressing for their families, because they followed a very sudden and quick deterioration that was unexpected, despite the cancer. It was agonisingly painful to try to imagine what John and Vincent must have gone through during their final hour, yet their families could not stop themselves from doing this over and over again. Six months after Vincent's sudden death, his sister-in-law Susan could not stop thinking about the fear Vincent must have felt as he was trying to wipe up the blood that poured from his mouth, trying to make one last desperate phone call. Susan was traumatised: 'I go to bed at night and I have that image in my head of him lying on the bed, propped up against the wall, with the phone in his hand.' My notes describe what John's mother and brothers told me six weeks after John died:

> *Margaret cannot stop herself from remembering her last conversation with John, the night before he died. She had been waiting for him to ring her, as he always did after watching Coronation Street: 'Did you see it?' 'Yes, I did.' When he still hadn't rung at 7.45pm, she rang him. His mobile rang for a long time before he answered it. He hadn't watched Coronation Street; he had been asleep. 'I just said, "Oh well, you have a good sleep, I'll speak to you in the morning."' Margaret laments, 'If only I'd known...'*
>
> *Margaret and her sons are full of angry questions. Why had he been so sleepy? Had he been given extra morphine? They are understandably furious at not being told that John had died in the morning; but they are also upset by knowing so little about what happened. I have been given some information by the nurses, and tell them as much as I know about the circumstances of John's death.*

Months later, their anger and distress was undiminished. Margaret agonised over and over again: 'If only I'd known... I should have been there. We should have been by his side. Not those bloody nurses.'

What is a 'good death'?

'Dying a good death' may seem like a contradiction in terms. Death constitutes unbearable loss. How can that ever be good? Yet there was a sense among the carers that they wanted the death to be as 'good' as it could be, and they had some ideas about the important components of such a 'good death'.

One aspect of a good death is *a sense of readiness.* 'I'm not ready for heaven yet,' John Davies said: 'There are still things I want to do.' But nine months later, his body ravaged by cancer, he was much more resigned. 'I've achieved everything... I am on my way to heaven.'

Others did not say as explicitly that they were close to death, but it was helpful and comforting for those around them if they seemed to accept their physical decline. Pete Carpenter, who had always been afraid of death, was remarkably calm throughout his illness. Sally Burnett told the hospice nurses that she was dying. Lily Lamb realised that she was staying in the hospice; her brother took this as a sign of understanding, which comforted him, even though she remained restless.

Many people spoke of their wish for the person to die *in familiar or safe surroundings with familiar people.* For some, this meant home: the carers of Pete Carpenter, Nick Ballard, Ursula Smith and Ben Edwards were passionate in their desire to keep them at home. However, other settings were possible. Sally and Lily were content at the hospice, and their families were happy, too. What seemed important was that people were in a place of safety, where their physical needs could be met and where close bonds with families and carers could be continued until the moment of death and beyond. This did not necessarily have to be at home (Tuffrey-Wijne 2009b).

Only John Davies openly acknowledged his impending death with me. The other people did not say anything to me about where they wanted to die. I did not feel I could ask them directly about dying, as I was bound by the ethical guidelines underpinning the Veronica Project not to introduce or intrude on such a sensitive topic without the person's agreement. As far as I could make out, they did not talk about it with anyone else.

However, it was clear that people's own ideas about a 'good place of death' could change over time. It would have been impossible for Lily Lamb to anticipate that she would rather be in a hospice than at home; yet that was what she actually preferred once she was admitted to the hospice: 'Stay here.' She did not want to go home. This was possibly influenced not only by her increased physical needs, but also by the fact that she, herself, never really saw her residential care home as 'home'. Similarly, both John Davies and Richard Horwood were content in a nursing home, something they could not have predicted even a few months beforehand. Circumstances change; the debilitating effects of cancer are difficult to imagine. People changed their minds as their condition changed.

The difficulty of knowing what a 'good death' would look like was further illustrated by John's thoughts on the best place to die. He had initially told me that he wanted to die in hospital, because he didn't want his family to have to witness it. Later, as we were preparing his story for publication, he asked me to change the text. 'I want to die at home with my mum,' he said. 'I've changed my mind about that.' There was ongoing tension between not wanting to be a burden, and wanting to be with loved ones; such tension was difficult, if not impossible, to resolve.

The third important component was *freedom from pain and anxiety.* Whether people were truly pain free could be difficult to assess; some were very good at hiding their physical and emotional pain. However, it seems that a number of people died in pain: Lily was never pain free; neither was Vincent; John's pain had become uncontrollable in his final days. Nick Ballard's pain could probably have been controlled, but Mary did not want him to have morphine until his very last days. Good pain control requires the input of skilled doctors and nurses: GPs or, if the pain is complex, palliative care teams. Several people did indeed have highly complex pain problems, a combination of physical and emotional pain that could not be controlled with medication alone. Only when families, support workers, doctors, nurses and other professionals worked together could the dying person benefit from as much physical and emotional support as was possible. This happened in some of the cases where people's dying lasted several days; but deaths that took people unawares, even though they had been very ill, were not fully supported.

Finally, it was clear that *the closest carers needed extensive support* if they were to experience a loved one's death as 'good'. They wanted to know exactly what was happening, or (if they could not be present) what had happened. They liked to have compassionate professionals around, who were competent in their support of the dying person, and aware of the carers' need for support and information. They seemed to need recognition of their grief, and they wanted to see that the person was treated with respect.

Bob and May did not mind that they weren't present at Lily's death; they accepted that they could not be there all the time, and were satisfied that the nurses did everything possible to keep Lily comfortable and to keep the family informed.

Being able to take time when someone died could help enormously. The support workers' distress at Pete Carpenter's death, when he was whisked away in an ambulance after attempted resuscitation, was partly because they wanted to be able to spend time with him after he died. In contrast, Mary said of Nick Ballard's death: 'When he died, he looked really peaceful. We did everything, washed him, laid him out, it was nice, you know?'

Funerals

Ursula Smith's funeral lasted half an hour and was attended by only five mourners. Pete Carpenter's funeral started with a wake the night before, full of story-telling, reminiscing and songs; the day of the funeral attracted hundreds of mourners who had travelled from all corners of England and beyond, and shifted from a deeply moving church service to a personalised cremation to drinks and cakes at the home where he had lived.

Funerals said something about the individuals who had died, but they said as much about the people they had left behind, their families, friends and care organisations, and the relationships between all these. They also reflected their culture. Vincent Sweeney came from an Irish Catholic family. After he died, his body was brought to the church the night before a requiem mass attended by large numbers of people.

Here are the descriptions of just two of the funerals, those of Dimas Ferreira and Sally Burnett, taken directly from my notes.

The funeral of Dimas Ferreira

> *I arrive at the church 15 minutes early. Mrs Lopez, Dimas' aunt, is standing outside with a few other people. She recognises me and shakes my hand warmly, thanking me for coming. I am impressed, later on, by the way she helps everyone and takes control, introducing people to each other (even me), and making sure everything is arranged properly. She has obviously organised the funeral. She tells me about Dimas' death, how she was with him when he died. Asked how it was, she says, thoughtfully, 'OK. It was OK.'*
>
> *Other people turn up: Dimas' father (living in Thailand) and brother (living elsewhere in the UK). Jason, the home manager, arrives. Apparently, several support workers are stuck in traffic. In the end, we go and sit in the church. It is a small gathering.*
>
> *Mrs Lopez asks the carers to sit on one side of the church, and family and friends on the other. This seems somewhat strange to me. Where should I sit? Where should his house mates sit, or the few carers from the past who have turned up? Are they carers or friends? Or even part of his family, having shared his home? When the coffin is brought in, there are 12 family members (all white) on one side, and about 12 support workers (mainly black) on the other. Later, a few more support workers arrive, with five people with*

learning disabilities, joining the 'black' side. I had planned to sit somewhere inconspicuous, but that is not really possible with such a small congregation.

Throughout the Catholic mass, the organ plays long hymns. Very few people are singing – at one hymn, nobody sings at all. There are other uncomfortable moments. A woman with learning disabilities sitting at the back makes loud noises, causing the support workers at the front to giggle; she is temporarily accompanied out of the church. Several times, the support workers look confused, clearly not familiar with the rituals of a Catholic mass.

I don't get much sense of Dimas' life, or of whether or not he is mourned. Mrs Lopez obviously cared. Some ex-support workers are chatting beforehand about how they used to take Dimas out, but then swiftly move on to discuss their own lives. The service seems impersonal. The only relief from this comes from two support workers who stand up to sing 'The Lord is my Shepherd' together; and from the priest – he hadn't met Dimas, but he tries to give a personalised address. He speaks of Dimas as someone with a child-like innocence, who didn't have the problems that we all have, such as cynicism. 'He didn't worry about the future, but took each day as it came. His life was simple: if you gave him love, he gave you love back. We should all try to be more like that.'

After the funeral service, people gather outside, waiting to go to the crematorium. I leave, and so do two people with learning disabilities and their support workers; we walk together for a bit. It is difficult to see how Dimas' death has affected them.

I cannot help wondering what the impact of Dimas' life has been on the people around him. What was his place in society? Will he be remembered?

The funeral of Sally Burnett

It is a cold, grey and drizzly day… People keep arriving, and it becomes clear that this is not the funeral of a person who lived an isolated or relationship-poor life. There is an eclectic mix of people from all abilities, all colours and all faiths. There are people in wheelchairs; I spot a Muslim scarf and a Sikh turban. Some people seemed to know Sally a long time ago, and have not necessarily kept in touch with her recently. School teachers and people from past clubs. I recognise the woman from Sally's dance class.

The hearse arrives, large, covered with flowers. I can see her Special Olympics medal on top of the coffin. There is Joy and her family. The funeral director comes up to us, asking us to come inside, 'Family first, then friends.' He asks us to share the booklets with the order of service. 'I have to say, there are more of you than we have booklets for.' Abba's 'Dancing Queen' plays. The chapel quickly fills up; in the end, there is standing room only. There must have been at least 150 people.

We all stand and fall silent as the coffin is carried in. It is a poignant moment. The family tribute paints a picture of Sally's life. Her disabilities are a strong part of it. How she was diagnosed with autism when she was very little, and how she briefly went into an institution. How it was said that she would never amount to much. How every milestone was a triumph: learning to walk, talk, read and write. How ('you wouldn't believe it now') she was initially frightened of going out, but overcame her fears, joined an athletics club and went on to win medals, even run for England. How proud she was to gain her independence when she moved into her own flat. How she always got involved in things. She loved dancing, and would be the first on the dance floor, the last to leave. She had 'an autistic gift for remembering dates. She could tell you what day of the week your birthday would fall in whatever year you asked her.' She loved holidays in the caravan, sitting at the seaside, watching the world go by. She loved her family, and would always keep an interest in them, whilst getting on with her own life. The tribute ends, 'Sally was a special needs person, and a very special person.' Sally's achievements are highlighted again in the tribute by her atheletics coaches, who describe her as 'an inspiration to young sports people'.

People all around me have been wiping their eyes, and more hankies come out as the curtains close at the committal. It is followed by a 'time of reflection' to the sound of Jason Donovan's 'Any Dream will Do'. One of the younger family members in the front row starts to sob loudly and inconsolably. Sally's sister goes round to comfort him. Other family members also weep, including Joy. Such crying is actually quite helpful in allowing others to cry, too. I feel the tears rolling down my own cheeks; all around me, people are reaching for their hankies...

I meet the hospice nurses on the train, and we talk a bit about Sally, about the way this funeral reflected her life. 'She couldn't walk,' says one of the nurses to the other, reflecting. 'All that running and dancing, and it was her legs, she couldn't walk...'

Reflecting on the funerals of people with learning disabilities

It became evident at the funerals that the people in the Veronica Project had a wide variety of people involved in their lives: families, paid carers and friends. This could be a time of coming together and celebrating someone's life, as in Sally's case; but it could also show the conflicts and tensions between families and support staff, particularly for those who lived in residential services. Who are the chief mourners? Who should carry the coffin, give a tribute, do the readings? Such issues could become painful, as it was at Dimas' funeral where the mourners were literally divided into two sections, and where the home manager later said angrily that the family should not have taken such a prominent part.

Most funerals were well attended, and most were very personal, with moving tributes and poignant readings. People were mourned and remembered, and their lives were celebrated. However, there was a strong insistence on the positive aspects of people's lives and characters, focusing on achievements and happiness. At times, this did not seem to measure up to the often painful lives people had led. This was most obvious when the celebrant had not known the person who had died. The priest at Dimas' funeral spoke of his 'child-like innocence', a person 'who didn't have the problems that we all have'. Nick Ballard, who was by no means an easy man and had certainly not had an easy life, was nevertheless described at his funeral as:

> 'A man who loved life. Someone who took life by the scruff of the neck and lived it to the full. Someone who was happy with his lot in life and made the most of it. The world does not have enough people like that.'

Most funerals in our society tend to give a positive view of the deceased and certainly avoid speaking ill of the dead. Mourners need comfort and reassurance, particularly if the last illness has been painful. The sometimes hidden feelings of profound pain and loss went unacknowledged at the funerals, but this failure to talk about painful lives at someone's funeral is probably not unusual. However, the determination to be positive about the lives of people with learning disabilities seemed to go beyond this. People's disabilities were mentioned, but the mourners then focused on how happy the person had been. In some cases, it sounded as if people with learning disabilities were happier because they were spared the pain of adult responsibility or of worrying about the complexities of life. Having listened to the people in the Veronica Project as carefully as I could, I found little resonance. Yes, there had been genuinely happy moments in their lives; people's lives were celebrated, and quite rightly so. But it sometimes seemed that mourners sought reassurance in people's smiles and their moments of joy, as if trying to confirm the idea that having learning disabilities is equivalent with being happy.

Grieving and remembering

Were the people with learning disabilities in the Veronica Project mourned after their deaths? Were they remembered? Did they leave a gaping hole in somebody's life? Did they leave a legacy?

These are important questions. As Stuart Todd points out, 'It is, perhaps, in death that one can begin to sum up the value of an individual's life' (Todd 2002, p.234). Here was a group of people who, on the whole, had not been made to feel that their lives were particularly important or valuable; Marion Prentice's mother had even been encouraged to think about her young child as already dead. Five people had spent much of their lives in institutional settings, segregated from society, only moving into ordinary neighbourhoods in recent decades. Apart from their bonds with family, most of the people with learning disabilities had not built many lasting relationships.

Grieving families

Family bonds continued to be important, even after people had died. The death of a son, a daughter, a brother or sister with learning disabilities constituted an irreplaceable loss. This is where the people with learning disabilities left a gap that could not be filled. Bereaved relatives cried when they talked of their special bond. This was true even for those who didn't have regular contact.

Marion Prentice's sister Sarah, who had not known about Marion's existence for a long time and who lived too far away to visit regularly, was devastated by Marion's death: 'I am finding it very difficult to come to terms with, I must admit.' She was distressed at the thought of Marion's difficult and lonely life, separated from her family and not regarded as a full member of society. She was particularly distressed at a remark from Marion's GP at the time of Marion's death:

> 'He said, "What do you expect, she's got Down's, she is old." That really upset me. They shouldn't just dismiss her like that.

> It was as if she was just seen as "Down's syndrome", not as an individual. What also upset me was that they put it on the death certificate: "Down's syndrome". As if she was just that. But you don't die of Down's syndrome, do you? You die of other things.'

Family members with learning disabilities were an important part of their relatives' lives, and it was upsetting if others did not recognise this.

Pete Carpenter's sister Joy experienced profound feelings of grief several years after he died: 'He was my only brother.' This resonated with Bob's feelings of loss: 'She was just Lily. She was my sister.'

John Davies' mother Margaret was so devastated by his death that it may well have accelerated her own death seven months later.

Vincent's sister-in-law Susan was in tears when she said:

> 'I miss him coming round. He always came on a Tuesday, and I would sort out his money for him. He was so proud of the money he'd managed to save. For the first time in his life. He said, now I've got money to go out and do what I like! In fact he had saved so much, his savings paid for the funeral… He had a sad life.'

Sally Burnett's stepmother Joy was not a person to wallow, and busied herself even more with the other relatives that needed her care and support. Her house was filled with memories. Sally looked out at her from photographs stuck onto the kitchen cupboards, surrounded by pictures of her siblings, nieces and nephews; Sally's watch hung over the framed photograph of her father. Two years after Sally's death, Joy said: 'She is always with me… I feel honoured that she was in my life. She enriched my life.'

It was profoundly moving to listen to these bereaved families. There was no doubt in my mind that here, at least, people lived on. They were still talked about. They would not be forgotten.

Support workers

I did not stay in contact with the support workers in the way I did with some of the families. In several cases (including Lily Lamb's), all the support workers who had been involved in someone's care had left when I contacted the residential care home a year later. In terms of mourning, it seemed that most service systems did not expect support workers to grieve. There was little structured support and recognition for feelings of loss, beyond the odd meeting to debrief.

After Dimas Ferreira's death, his home manager Jason said that his staff had found it all quite difficult; he was planning to have a meeting to discuss this. 'Hopefully we'll be able to move on after that.'

The only home I stayed in regular contact with was Pete Carpenter's. This home had an explicitly Christian ethos. There was a culture of remembering the dead, with annual rituals involving both support workers and residents reflecting on their own personal losses and on the residents who had died. Several years after his death, Pete Carpenter had taken a firm place in the history of this group of homes; his story was remembered, his songs were still sung, and his painting hung on the wall of his old home.

Not having followed up many of the support workers, it is impossible to say how the death of a resident affected the staff. Mostly, support workers and health care staff remembered the people who had died with affection. Those who felt bereft, such as Mary, busied themselves with their work, not focusing on the impact of the death on their own lives. The staff had been touched by the people who had died, and their future work may well have been influenced by them; but for the support workers in the Veronica Project that I kept in contact with, the loss seemed less profound than for the families.

The impact of the deaths on people's friends was even more difficult to assess. I did not focus on their friends and peers, and did not follow them up. The friends of people with learning disabilities have not been given much attention by other researchers and clinicians either.

Leaving a legacy

Many of us want to leave a legacy. We find solace in knowing that we can pass on the essence of ourselves, through our children, our work, our achievements, our actions. We want to leave our footprints behind when we die.

Loved ones, too, are comforted by knowing that the person who has died somehow lives on; that the world is a different place, a better place, because of the person who has now died.

Leaving a legacy was important for several people. John Davies was the most articulate and driven in wanting to leave something behind. His contribution to the Veronica Project was one thing; the DVD he recorded for his mother was another: 'So that when I've gone to heaven she's got something to remember me by,' he said. He was explicit in naming others who should also receive a copy.

People's legacies consisted mostly of the memories they left behind with their families. As Bob said, 'She will always be there.' It was more difficult to assess the legacy of those who had little to leave and few people to miss them, like Ursula Smith or Dimas Ferreira.

When people were offered help to leave a legacy, however small, they took it. John set to work making silk scarves in the hospice day centre, and had a list of people in his mind that he wanted to give them to as a way of saying thank you, including members of his family and his cancer nurse. Lily painted a special plate. They may have enjoyed such creative activities throughout their lives – Lily was an expert at silk painting because of her many day centre classes – but John's scarves and Lily's plate, made during the last months of their lives, seemed to be particularly imbued with meaning.

The desire to make a difference and leave something behind was one reason why many people and their families were very keen to take part in the Veronica Project. For the people with learning disabilities, it was the chance to have their stories recorded and published that captured their imagination. For their families, it was the strong desire that others should learn from it, that the experience of their loved one could be of benefit to other people with learning disabilities. They wanted the world to recognise the value of people like Marion, Sally and Lily. 'There is still prejudice,' one of the relatives said. 'There is still discrimination.'

Summary

Dying

- Ten people died during the Veronica Project.
- The process of dying was varied, and probably no different from deaths in the general population. Some people deteriorated

gradually, with a dying process lasting several days; others died quickly and unexpectedly.

- Death always came as a shock to the closest carers, who often felt deeply distressed. They remembered the final hours vividly and kept going over it in their minds, sometimes full of regret.

- Carers saw a 'good death' as a death:

  - for which the person was, in some ways, 'ready'
  - in familiar or safe surroundings with familiar people – this did not necessarily have to be at home
  - free from pain and anxiety
  - where the closest carers received intensive support.

Funerals

- People's funerals varied widely, and reflected their social and cultural backgrounds.
- People were mourned and remembered, and their lives were celebrated.
- There was a tendency to paint a positive, 'happy' picture of the people with learning disabilities at their funerals.

Grieving and remembering

- The people with learning disbilities were grieved for by their families. Their deaths left a gaping hole in their relatives' lives.

- Most learning disability services did not expect support workers to grieve. There was little support and recognition for feelings of loss. Some support workers did feel the loss and were deeply upset.

- The impact of the death of people with learning disabilities on their friends has not received sufficient attention.
- Several people wanted to leave a legacy. The participants and their families felt that their contribution to this book would be a lasting and positive legacy; they wanted others to learn from their experiences.

CHAPTER 9

Learning Lessons

Thinking about the people in the Veronica Project, I often wondered whether their experiences were as good as they could have been. Could, or should, things have been different? How can we support people with learning disabilities who are ill? How can we ensure that the end of someone's life is not more difficult than it has to be?

For all the people whose stories have been told in this book, there were aspects of care and support that could have been better. Some of the difficulties could and should be addressed; for example, the ignorance and assumptions of some staff about the needs and capacities of people with learning disabilities clearly needs attention. But maybe some of the difficulties were unavoidable. There is no way of making cancer and dying easy. Cancer can be a devastating, ravaging and messy illness. Even the best plans and the best intentions cannot always prevent a distressing outcome, simply because cancer can bring unexpected and sudden changes. There is also no way of preventing families and carers from experiencing a wide range of emotions, including feelings of guilt, anger and distress.

Even for the people whose cancers were diagnosed early and who were successfully treated, those treatments were invasive, exhausting and sometimes shocking. Pauline never forgot the 'black sausage' the surgeon removed from her breast; Amanda remembered times when she wanted to join her mother who had died two decades earlier.

For those who didn't survive, the process of gradually losing strength was often very hard for their families and carers to witness. Several people had to cope with the loss of their ability to walk. Most people suffered pain; for some, this was never totally relieved. Carers changed the bed sheets when people became incontinent, and helped people up from the floor where they had laid down weak and exhausted. Coping with cancer and dying meant coping with worry, loss and grief, but it also meant coping with an often unanticipated and relentless process of physical deterioration. How can such grim facts ever make for a good experience?

In fact, many of my experiences with the people in the Veronica Project were positive, even uplifting. It wasn't all difficult. There was something good and inspiring in every person's story. It is those positive aspects that can be most helpful when we contemplate how end-of-life support could be improved for others. Might it be possible to think of a situation where everything that went well for the people in this book was combined, and where someone with learning disabilities was supported in his or her cancer journey and in dying in the best possible way? In this final chapter I will contemplate what such support would look like. It is based on my assessment of what the people with learning disabilities in this book found important and helpful.

What did people want and need?

To be diagnosed in good time

Sometimes, it is simply not possible to diagnose cancer at a stage where it can be cured. If people do not complain or show any signs or symptoms, it may well be too late by the time their carers notice that anything is wrong. Sometimes, changes in behaviour that are symptomatic of an underlying physical cause are so subtle, and could indicate such a wide range of possible causes, that it is almost unavoidable that the diagnosis is not made immediately. Yet receiving the cancer diagnosis was important; even in those situations where the person was already terminally ill, having a diagnosis meant that support could be put into place.

Some families or carers were alert and sensitive to changes in behaviour or to complaints that may indicate that someone is not well. Lily's family knew that her complaints of pain should be taken seriously, because she never usually complained. Marion's key worker wasn't convinced that her breast cancer had gone, because she 'just wasn't herself'. When Ursula started having falls, Mary took her to the doctor straight away, insisting on tests. Dimas' support workers were persistent and swift, taking him back to the doctor when they noticed that the lump on his neck had grown, even though the hospital had sent him home the night before and told the carers not to worry.

When people went to seek medical advice, the doctor then had to act. Some people were sent for tests immediately. A speedy reaction from Marion's hospital meant that her cancer could be treated successfully.

To receive treatment and care that is based on their own wishes, and on 'best interest'

Being involved in treatment decisions helped people to cope with the treatment. Amanda knew that the alternative, not having the treatment, would lead to a bleak outcome. Pauline chose radiotherapy over chemotherapy. Even those whose cognitive abilities were more limited could often understand the reasons for treatment and choose it: Marion didn't want a messy breast and underwent a mastectomy.

When someone lacked the capacity to make treatment choices, others had to decide what was best. The decision was more likely to be balanced and truly based on the person's best interest if it was made by a group of people, not just an individual carer or doctor. A 'best interest meeting' for Ben incorporated the doctor's knowledge of likely treatment outcomes; Yanna's intimate knowledge of Ben's usual way of coping with hospitals, tests and treatments; and his family's love and desire to do what was best for him.

To be free of pain and other symptoms

Almost all cancer patients will experience a range of uncomfortable and unpleasant symptoms. Without prompt and skilled care, these symptoms can dominate the patient's life.

Day-to-day carers, whether they were family or residential care staff, could not be expected to have the necessary knowledge to control pain and other symptoms such as nausea, constipation or a dry mouth. They needed the input of experts to advise them, to prescribe the necessary medication and to reassure and support them in giving it. Such help came from doctors and nurses, for example, palliative care nurses visiting the home. John's hospice had developed guidelines about supporting patients with learning disabilities; they accepted early referrals and visited regularly even when everyone was coping well, recognising that it was important and might take more time to build up trusting relationships.

Some people in the Veronica Project only became pain free when such outside professionals were able to act. For Nick, this didn't happen until the final few days of his illness, when the community palliative care nurse convinced Mary that he should have morphine. A few weeks earlier, hospital staff had given him a dose of morphine that had transformed him back into his old self.

Lily's symptoms were complex and could not be controlled at home, despite the best efforts of the care staff, the district nurses and the community palliative care nurse. She needed the expertise of hospice staff 24 hours a day. Lily herself realised this, and asked to move into a place where there were doctors and nurses: 'I should be in hospital.' Thankfully, for her, a hospice place was available and offered.

To have dignity

Having dignity meant not being patronised, being spoken to and not ignored; being helped when help was needed and allowed to manage yourself when it was not. I sometimes had to stop myself from helping Pauline as she struggled to make me a cup of tea in the kitchen of her new flat.

Pete's carers gave him dignity by constantly including him in conversation. Here is what happened when Pete's palliative care nurse came to assess him at home:

> *The nurse asks Ramesh* [home manager]*: 'Does his family visit him?' Ramesh is very good at answering her whilst including Pete: 'Your sister Daphne comes to visit you sometimes, doesn't she? A couple of times a year. And you used to visit her at her house, but now you don't – you don't like the travel.'*

Looking and smelling nice was important to several people. Sometimes this could be as simple as families or carers bringing someone's own clothes into hospital, but sometimes it needed more effort, even expertise. The smell of cancerous wounds or colostomy bags was sometimes hard to disguise, but it was not impossible. This was evident during a visit to John at the hospice two months before he died.

> *John is sitting in an armchair, feet raised, by the window of his hospice room, whilst two nurses finish off making his bed. He looks well cared for, with well-fitting clothes that cover up any hint of abdominal wounds or bags; for the first time since I've known him, there is absolutely no smell. Apart from the fact that he is sitting on a pressure-relieving cushion and occasionally winces when he shifts in his chair, he would not be particularly ill to the eyes of the uninitiated. I realise only now that the physical care in hospital (or at home, for that matter) 'could be better'.*

To have adequate equipment and space

Many people had difficulty walking up the stairs. Richard was relieved when he finally got a chair lift. Nick loved his new en-suite bedroom, specially adapted for him on the ground floor. Homes that were able to offer someone an accessible room were best placed to accommodate a very ill resident.

Sometimes it wasn't possible to put the necessary resources in place; either there simply wasn't the physical possibility of adapting the home, or there wasn't enough time. In such cases, it was sometimes better for the person to move somewhere else. Lily liked the hospice because here she had the space for a wheelchair and a hoist that took her straight into the bath.

Sometimes, the staff in the residential care home bought the necessary equipment themselves, because they could not wait. A wheelchair for Ursula; an armchair for Pete. Very few of the teams made use of the support of an outside professional who might be able to help them to plan ahead and co-ordinate resources: for example, a community learning disability nurse, a community palliative care nurse or a district nurse.

To receive as much information as they want, in a way they can understand

Some people could understand explanations when they were given clearly and simply. Amanda wanted as much information as possible and was able to ask for it: 'What is lymphoma?'

Vincent was very happy after his hospital doctor managed to explain to him in simple words what was happening with his cancer. Previous consultations, when he could not understand either the doctor's language or the X-ray images, had upset and angered him.

Some people could not understand words alone. Marion's carers were the only ones who made extensive use of pictures when they explained to her what was happening. They used the expertise of the community learning disability nurse, who made a personalised book for Marion, explaining step by step what would happen during her mammogram. Unlike the residential care staff, the community learning disability team had hospital contacts and could gain knowledge of the medical aspects of Marion's care, which enabled the nurse to help both Marion and her team of carers prepare for her tests and treatment.

People wanted honesty without being overwhelmed. It was helpful for Sally, early in her illness, to be told that she was 'living with cancer'. When she finally said 'I think I'm dying,' just a few weeks before her death, her stepmother and the hospice staff didn't deny it. The few months beforehand, when her family and staff told her that she was doing OK and would be able to go back home when she was better, were confusing and possibly upsetting.

To have a degree of control over their lives

Lily said she liked making decisions. Vincent wanted to stay at home, where he could be in control.

Control over major choices, such as whether or not to have radiotherapy or where to die, was obviously important. The hospice team gave John a choice about going into a nursing home; he could even choose which one, having visited two different homes. Likewise, Richard said that he should go into a nursing home, and decided to move to a different nursing home when he didn't like the first one. Both these men were happy in the home they chose and continued to make their own choices about what they did with their time. The sensitive and understanding staff did not stop Richard going 'out and about'.

Ben showed that he wanted to stay at his residential care home by his clear pride and love of his bedroom. This convinced his residential care team that they should do everything possible to support him at home.

But making choices did not only mean major choices; it also meant relatively minor choices, such as whether to walk about or to sit and rest. Nick did not have much control over his life, but when he did, he was clearly happier. Unlike most of the day centre staff who stuck to rigid rules and routines, his day centre key worker was sensitive to his wishes.

> *Nick spots the painting and wants to join in. He signs 'apron'. His supporter comes in and says that he has to come out, he is meant to be cooking. He ignores her, and when she has left, walks over to the drawer full of aprons. He picks one out, puts it on, and asks me to tie it up at the back (I oblige). His key worker comes in at this point, and is far more relaxed, far less directive: 'He just loves painting. Oh, OK, Nick, you can do a little bit before you carry on with your cooking.' And to the supporter who drops back in: 'It's fine, he is here for a while.' Nick happily sets about the paint work.*

To have contact with their families

Most of the care homes made a concerted effort to welcome people's families. Yanna's understanding of the important place of his brother in Ben's life meant that she telephoned him immediately when she felt Ben was very unwell. Ben's brother came; Ben died the next morning. Pete's sister Daphne found it too difficult to visit Pete when he was very ill, but his carers always let her know what was happening.

Positive family contact needed to be supported throughout the people's lives, not just when they were dying. It was only because Yanna had worked hard at helping Ben re-establish contact with his family that they were able to be with him in his final weeks. Sometimes, it simply wasn't possible to include family. Nick's stepmother wrote to Mary, telling her that she wanted to receive no further news about him.

Some people's families had always featured strongly in their lives, and this became even more important when they were ill. John, Vincent, Lily and Sally were all very clear about their love of their families and their need for family support. Their families needed to be included and receive support themselves. Lily's brother and sister-in-law were kept up to date by the hospice staff. The staff met with them frequently, both formally and informally. They could visit Lily at any time of the day or night.

To have contact with their friends

John, Vincent and Amanda kept in contact with friends when they were ill. They could manage their friendships independently by making phone calls or sending text messages, and most of their friends could visit them without support. Others needed help to be with their friends. Pete's support workers took him to his day centre where he could sit among his friends, even when he was very ill. However, very few friends with learning disabilities were helped to visit the ill person during the last weeks or months of life.

To have carers who are well supported, both practically and emotionally

The burden of care could be overwhelming for families and support workers. Several people with learning disabilities showed that they were acutely aware of this, and that they worried about it.

Residential care services that planned ahead were more likely to have teams that felt supported. The director of Ben Edwards' residential care service explained, 'We try to give the homes some extra support as soon as someone is diagnosed.' The director of the group of homes where Pete lived called a meeting the week after his diagnosis, involving his direct carers and his sister. They discussed his physical and emotional care and identified sources of support, including the palliative care team and district nurses. They also discussed what to tell Pete, and how to support the team.

Sometimes, carers needed to be shown how to cope with the physical needs of the ill person. John's family learned from the nurses how to change the dressings of his wounds, which was a complex task. Mary's experiences when Ursula was in hospital, just a day before Ursula died, showed clearly that she needed the nurses' support. She said:

> 'Ursula wanted to walk to the toilet but she was not allowed, because her breathing is so bad. So in the end they just gave me the bedpan, but I don't know how to do a bedpan. I can't

> lift Ursula. I was trying to lift her up onto it, but it was difficult, so then the bed got wet… And then they just left me to wash her. A nurse came, but she saw me and she said, "Oh good, you're doing it," and left. In the end the sister helped me, she saw me struggling and then she helped me to make her comfortable. We washed her and changed the sheets.'

District nurses were ideally placed to teach daily carers about basic nursing tasks such as regular mouth care, or how to change the sheets with the person still in bed; but such sharing of skills rarely happened, and the carers didn't ask. They sometimes lurched from crisis to crisis. Pete's carers improvised when they found him on the floor, and they panicked when he suddenly became incontinent in bed.

Often, preventing carers from becoming exhausted meant that they needed extra resources, extra staff. Lily's home manager didn't know how she would cope with Lily's physical care needs when there was only one member of staff on duty, but a week later she looked much more relaxed. The senior managers had allocated more staff to the home. Sadly, such extra resources were not always available. Putting in extra support workers at the end of life needs not only a policy commitment but also extra money.

Emotional support for families and carers was important, too. This needed to include support from managers and outside professionals such as hospice teams or an understanding GP. Carers needed recognition of the emotional burden they carried, the worry, fear and grief inherent in supporting someone who was dying. Yanna was hugely appreciative of the regular phone calls from her senior managers, offering her a chance to talk through her worries, as well as the knowledge that she could ask for extra resources if needed. Almost without exception, carers needed to know that there was 'someone at the end of the line', someone they could ask for help.

People who were ill and dying were best supported if their carers were well supported. Carers were best supported if there was active involvement from a range of agencies. GPs who didn't mind being called upon frequently. District nurses who visited the home and provided practical nursing support. Palliative care nurses who gave advice on end-of-life care, including symptom control. Community learning disability teams who helped with communication, planning and accessing resources.

Each of these agencies brings a different and necessary skill. The pooling of such skills, where the different agencies recognise that they can and must benefit from the input of others, can be extremely successful. There were no clear examples of such collaboration within the Veronica Project, but I have heard many positive stories from others, for example, a learning disability nurse going onto a hospital ward to teach the staff about communication. One palliative care nurse wrote in a questionnaire survey:

> I worked in partnership with the learning disabilities team. They assessed the patient's change of behaviour and interpreted what it meant. I provided the symptom control advice and altered the medication accordingly. Increase in aggressive behaviour [was] concluded to be an increase in pain. It was a very successful partnership. (Tuffrey-Wijne *et al.* 2008, p.286)

To have carers who love them

Without Mary's deep affection and genuine care for both Nick and Ursula, their illness and dying would have been much more difficult for them. Sally knew that she could rely on her stepmother Joy to be with her whenever she needed her.

Most people had one or more carers who truly loved them, and who would do anything to support them. Such loving carers could be relatives or paid staff. They were usually a constant presence during the person's illness. Many paid carers ignored the boundaries of shift patterns and job descriptions, and often went well beyond the call of duty.

The ability to show genuine affection, warmth and empathy cannot be captured in a carers' training session, yet it was obvious from the experiences of the people in the Veronica Project that 'love' mattered. It made the illness bearable.

The danger for carers who love the people they support is that their emotional commitment is unrecognised, unsupported and possibly even disapproved of. Such carers should be strongly supported, both practically and emotionally. They should not carry their burden alone. Burn-out is much more likely if carers feel that only they can be relied upon to provide support; that only they can understand the person's needs; that it is essential they are available 24 hours a day, seven days a week. Some carers would not feel able to share their caring role, even if that was made possible. Mary said, 'Even if I had more staff, I would still want to do it all myself.' However, it could make a real difference to have someone – usually an outside professional or a senior manager – who could offer carers at least a sympathetic listening ear. Their love – and their grief – should be openly allowed; it should not be disenfranchised.

To be allowed to be sad as well as happy

Nobody told John to cheer up when he prepared for the recording of his DVD, said, 'I love you, Mum,' into the microphone, and cried. The cheering came afterwards, when John himself grinned in delight at his achievement and was given a large bunch of flowers by staff from the hospice and theatre. The memory of that day, with the tears as well as the flowers and smiles, inspired and comforted him until he died.

Vincent could ring his friend Frank at any time to complain about his life and illness. Lily's brother and sister-in-law were able to sit and stay with her for long periods, holding her hand and massaging her legs, even when she looked deeply unhappy. They always gave her simple and honest answers. She needed them.

The exhortation of many staff and families to be happy and smiley, even when people were very ill, did not help people with learning disabilities to come to terms with their illness and impending death. People who were allowed to be sad as well as happy seemed to be able to be more fully themselves. They did not wallow in their sadness; they were still able to have happy or contented moments; but they also used the support others could give, even if that was just a supportive presence.

To 'keep going' with what they enjoy

John kept singing; Richard kept walking; Pete kept 'working', even if that meant simply being present in his day centre; Ben kept buying videos.

Many people were able to keep their favourite routines and activities going, even when they were very ill. The carers were impressed by people's dogged determination to keep going, and tried hard to accommodate it.

To be cared for, and to die, in a place where they feel safe and loved

It was difficult for people to spend their final days in a place that was unfamiliar and frightening. Dimas and Ursula did not want to be in hospital; they were unhappy during the time leading up to their deaths.

People wanted to be in a place where they could be looked after in comfort. For some, home was the most comfortable and safe environment; but others, such as Lily, Sally and John, realised that they could not be cared for properly at home, and preferred to be in a hospice or a nursing home.

People felt safe if they understood the routines, knew the people who cared for them and felt understood by them, and – most important of all – could be with the people they loved. This was most easily achieved if the person stayed at home, as happened for Pete, Nick and Ben; but being at home was not a prerequisite for 'a good death'. It was possible for carers in other settings to be sensitive to people's needs, to pick up their preferred ways of communicating, and to create a safe and predictable environment. The staff at Lily's hospice were a clear example of this.

To look back on their lives

All the people in the Veronica Project who could speak spent some time talking about the past: their relationships, the things that had happened. This was not simply because I asked them: they seemed keen to tell me, keen to reflect.

People were able to reflect on their lives in different ways. Having a researcher who listened to their stories was one of them. The families of both Lily and Sally brought an array of photographs and other mementoes into the hospice, which enabled staff and visitors to talk to them about some of the events and people that had shaped their lives. A member of staff who had worked with Pete in the past and who was a gifted musician came to see him a few times during Pete's last weeks of life. To Pete's delight, she sang him songs from the past, including songs Pete remembered from his childhood.

Nobody in the Veronica Project had a 'life story book', often used with people with learning disabilities services: an account of the person's life, including mementoes, stories and memories of past events and relationships. For people who have no access to musicians or a store of photographs, putting together such a book could be a good way to reflect on their lives.

To leave a legacy

People left a legacy in a variety of ways. Some legacies were tangible, like this book, people's photo albums and John's recordings – including not just his DVD, but all the songs he recorded on CD during the past decade. Other legacies consisted mostly of the indelible memories left behind with those who loved them. People wanted to be remembered. Some people said explicitly that they wanted their experiences to help others. People could be helped to create tangible memorials, for example, through craft projects or through putting together a life story book.

Conclusion

Most of the important aspects of people's care that I have described in this chapter would probably not be any different for people without learning disabilities. Being diagnosed in good time, having control over your life and illness, being pain free, receiving adequate information, being with loved ones, having a well-supported team of competent carers, being able to express emotions, being somewhere you can feel safe, being able to reflect on your life and leave a legacy – who would not want these things if they were ill and dying?

But what has struck me throughout the Veronica Project is how much support and sensitivity people with learning disabilities need for the end of their lives to be as good as they can possibly be, given the circumstances.

It would be wonderful if people with learning disabilities who are dying did not have to suffer from their carers' lack of knowledge or lack of sensitivity, or from lack of resources, on top of the suffering inherent in their illness. And it would be wonderful if carers and families could look back without too much guilt or reproach, cherishing memories of the final months, confident that everyone did everything possible to help the person cope with his or her illness and to ease that person's dying.

What is clear from all the stories in this book is that families, carers and professionals can make a real difference. Even one person can make a positive difference to the experience of someone with learning disabilities who is dying of cancer. However, it is also clear that people need each other. Even the most dedicated carer cannot do everything alone. Each person involved in the end-of-life support of someone with learning disabilities has an important contribution to make.

I hope this book helps readers to reflect with an open mind on the stories of people with learning disabilities that they know, and learn from them: the positive as well as the not-so-positive. Such learning is one of the tributes we can make to people with learning disabilities who have died. They leave a legacy through the way they have changed us and our perceptions, the way they have made us more sensitive and understanding.

This book is a starting point. We have only just begun the important task of listening to people with learning disabilities who are ill and dying, and there is still much work to be done. I hope that this book motivates other researchers to undertake further studies. And I hope that the experiences of the people in this book will help families, carers and other professionals to be confident and inspired in their support of people with learning disabilities at the end of their lives.

Listening to Pete, Dimas, John, Lily, Nick, Richard, Vincent, Marion, Pauline, Sally, Ben, Ursula and Amanda, it was clear to me that they would leave something of huge importance through the writing of this book. They showed me the value of their lives, and in doing so, they showed the value of the lives of all people with learning disabilities.

That is a legacy, indeed.

APPENDIX 1

The People in this Book

For ease of reference, here is an overview of the people who took part in the Veronica Project. All names have been changed, with the exception of Amanda Cresswell and John Davies who asked not to be anonymous.

Nick Ballard (56)

Nick had Down's syndrome with severe/profound learning disabilities. He had no hearing and no speech, using sounds and hand signs to communicate. He was admitted to a large hospital for people with learning disabilities in childhood, and now lived in a staffed residential care home with seven other residents. He attended a large day centre five days a week. There was no family contact. He was very close to **Mary**, his home manager.

Nick was diagnosed with advanced **cancer of the bladder**. He received no cancer treatments. He died at home 15 months after diagnosis, supported by Mary. Ursula Smith also lived in this home and was diagnosed with end-stage cancer six months after Nick's death.

Sally Burnett (45)

Sally had mild/moderate learning disabilities and autism. She did not initiate much conversation, but her understanding was good. She was very close to her stepmother **Joy**, who had married her father when Sally was in her teens. Sally lived alone with some family support, having previously lived in the parental home. She had a job at a supermarket and an active social life, and had once won a medal in the Special Olympics.

Sally had lived with **cancer of the bowel** for five years, coping well with her colostomy bag. The cancer had spread to the liver, lung and spine. Sally died in a hospice three months after a sudden deterioration. She desperately wanted to go back to her flat during her final months.

Pete Carpenter (66)

Pete had severe learning disabilities. He spoke in simple words and short sentences. He had many enthusiasms, including bikes, steam trains, jazz, and men in overalls working in the street. Pete grew up in the family home, and lived there until he was in his early forties and his parents died. His sister **Daphne** was his closest relative. Pete now lived in a staffed residential care home with two other residents. His home manager was **Ramesh**. Pete had many friends.

Pete was diagnosed with **cancer of the lung**, spread to the throat. The cancer was advanced; there was no treatment, and his prognosis was short. He died at his residential care home two months later.

Amanda Cresswell (36)

Amanda had mild learning disabilities and was very articulate. She had a job as an advocate for people with learning disabilities, and had previously worked as an actor. She had lived with foster carers since her mother died when she was in her early teens, but after her cancer treatments she moved into her own flat with some support from a carer.

Amanda was diagnosed with **lymphoma** five years ago. She went through a series of intensive treatments, and is now, it is hoped, free of cancer. Since taking part in the Veronica Project, Amanda has taken the initiative to publish her cancer story (Cresswell and Tuffrey-Wijne 2008). She has appeared in an education video for cancer professionals, and has spoken publicly about her cancer experiences in an effort to educate health care staff about the needs of people with learning disabilities.

John Davies (44)

John had mild learning disabilities. He was sociable and very articulate. He grew up with his mother **Margaret** and his brothers. He moved away as a young adult, living on the street, in hostels and eventually in his own flat. He loved music and singing, and worked as a volunteer with a performing arts centre for people with disabilities.

John was diagnosed with **cancer of the penis** after hiding his symptoms for many months. He had radical surgery, but the cancer returned, spreading widely in his abdominal area. John moved back to his mother's flat. He was often in hospital, where he received chemotherapy. He later went into a hospice and then a nursing home, where he died 18 months after diagnosis. His mother, whom John had been very close to, died six months later.

Pauline Deweert (56)

Pauline had mild/moderate learning disabilities. She had good understanding, and spoke clearly. She lived with her mother, but after her cancer treatments she moved into her own flat with on-site support staff.

Pauline was diagnosed with **cancer of the breast** five years ago. She had a lumpectomy followed by radiotherapy, and started taking Tamoxifen. She is now, it is hoped, free of cancer, but she remains somewhat fearful that the cancer will return.

Ben Edwards (44)

Ben had Down's syndrome and severe/profound learning disabilities. His speech was limited and difficult to understand. Ben lived with family until the age of 13, when he moved into a long-stay hospital for people with learning disabilities. He now lived in a residential care home with six other residents. His room was full of videos, mostly bought at charity shops. Ben was close to his long-term manager **Yanna**. He had re-established contact with his family, and he loved being with them.

Ben was diagnosed with **cancer of the testicles** five years ago, and received radiotherapy and chemotherapy. He went for regular checks at the hospital. After a gradual deterioration, Ben collapsed at home and was taken to hospital, where his life support machine was switched off soon afterwards.

Dimas Ferreira (47)

Dimas had severe/profound learning disabilities, and no speech. His understanding was limited to simple concepts. Dimas was abandoned by his parents in childhood, and lived in a hospital for people with learning disabilities, where his grandmother visited occasionally. His aunt **Mrs Lopez** took over these visits 14 years ago. Dimas moved into a staffed residential care home around the same time.

When his carers found a lump on his neck, Dimas was diagnosed with **cancer of unknown origin**, spread to the lymph nodes. No treatments were given. Dimas died in hospital ten months after the diagnosis. He hated hospitals.

Richard Horwood (64)

Richard had mild learning disabilities. He was articulate, but never wanted to talk for long. He had suffered from depression for decades. He spent most of his life moving between the parental home and institutional care, including a psychiatric hospital and a residential care home for people with learning disabilities. He now lived in his own flat with his friend **Charlie**, supported by social care staff. Richard loved walking, and often wandered into town, stopping at the café for lunch. A few times each week, he dropped into a large day centre for people with learning disabilities.

Richard was diagnosed with **cancer of the lung** that could not be treated. He remained fiercely independent throughout his illness, but when he became weaker, he moved into a nursing home at his own request. Although he was terminally ill, he was still active four years after the cancer diagnosis.

Lily Lamb (55)

Lily had mild/moderate learning disabilities. Her understanding was good, but her speech was hard to understand, which made her self-conscious. She lived with her parents until 15 years ago, when she moved into a staffed residential care home shared with five other residents. She was very close to her brother **Bob** and his wife **May**, and still saw the family as her real 'home'. Lily liked to do things well, and enjoyed having her own tasks and doing proper work in an office.

Lily was diagnosed with advanced **cancer of the stomach** which had spread to the bones. She was in much pain, and the home was unable to support her. She was moved into a hospice, where she died five months after diagnosis.

Marion Prentice (61)

Marion had Down's syndrome and severe/profound learning disabilities. Her understanding was limited, and she spoke in short sentences that were difficult to understand. When she was a baby, she went into a long-stay hospital for people with learning disabilities. She now lived in a staffed residential care home, together with several friends from the long-stay hospital. Her younger sister **Sarah**, who didn't know of Marion's existence for many years, now visited regularly.

Marion was diagnosed with **cancer of the breast**. She had a mastectomy and was thought to be cured of cancer. She found it difficult to go through hospital procedures, including mammograms, and needed careful preparation for this. Marion was later admitted to a nursing home with probable dementia, where she died of heart failure.

Ursula Smith (65)

Ursula had severe/profound learning disabilities. She had had mental health symptoms since childhood, including hallucinations and self-harm. She had lived in a long-stay hospital for people with learning disabilities, and moved into a staffed residential care home 18 years ago. Nick Ballard also lived in the home, which was managed by **Mary**. Ursula had no family. She spent most of her days sitting quietly in her chair.

Ursula was diagnosed with **cancer of the breast** 14 years previously, and had a lumpectomy. She was symptom free until six months after Nick Ballard died, when cancer was found in her bones. She had a dose of radiotherapy to control her pain. Ursula stayed at home. She went into hospital three months later, and died there.

Vincent Sweeney (47)

Vincent had mild learning disabilities. He had an easy manner and liked friendly chats. He grew up with his family. As an adult, he had lived in various hostels, including hostels for people with alcohol dependency. He had moved into his own flat a year before the cancer diagnosis, receiving little outside support. He was proud of his flat, and said he no longer drank. He loved his job at a local council office. Vincent was close to his sister-in-law **Susan**, who often helped him, and his brother **Donald**. He had several other siblings. His elderly mother lived some distance away.

Vincent was diagnosed with **cancer of the lung**. He had chemotherapy and radiotherapy. He started attending the hospice day centre. Vincent always felt very lonely and frightened. He died suddenly at home, alone, two and a half years after the diagnosis.

APPENDIX 2

Methods

This section describes the methodology used in the Veronica Project. It will be useful to those readers who want to assess the rigour of the research described in this book, and those who are interested in replicating or building on the study in some way.

Defining 'learning disabilities'

First of all, it is useful to explain what criteria we used under the heading 'learning disabilities' in assessing whether or not someone was eligible to participate in the Veronica Project.

The definition of 'learning disabilities' includes three aspects: 'the presence of a significantly reduced ability to understand new or complex information, to learn new skills (impaired intelligence), with a reduced ability to cope independently (reduced social functioning), which started before adulthood, with a lasting effect on development' (Department of Health 2001a, p.14). The initial research protocol stated that participants had to fall within the ICD-10 definition of 'mental retardation' (i.e. learning disability), which indicates an IQ of below 70 and impairment of a range of skills (World Health Organisation 1992).

In practice it was not possible to be sure whether people met these criteria. Only one of the participants had his IQ recorded in his notes. Whilst the presence of learning disability was undisputed for those with more severe cognitive impairments, it was more difficult to assess in those with less pronounced cognitive impairments. I therefore adopted a 'social systems perspective' as the main criterion for determining whether people could be said to have learning disabilities and were therefore eligible to participate in the Veronica Project. This followed the practice of other researchers, such as Booth and Booth in their study of parents with learning disabilities, who state that 'the only practical decision rule we could follow was to select parents who at some time in their lives, not necessarily currently, had been in receipt of health, education or social services specifically intended for people with learning difficulties' (Booth and Booth 1994a, p.416).

I was occasionally asked whether some participants really did have learning disabilities, and the answer was not always straightforward. For example, in the case of John Davies, I was unable to establish with certainty past use of learning disability services when I recruited him into the Veronica Project. The words 'Learning Disabilities' appeared in his medical notes; most of the staff supporting John felt that he had learning disabilities. At our first meeting, I asked him whether he himself thought he had learning disabilities. He said that he did, 'but it is in my legs, not in my head'. As it emerged later in the study, having the label of learning disabilities often affects people's experiences; it could well be that this is the case even if the label is wrong.

The lack of stated IQ or skills assessment meant it was difficult to make clear demarcations between those with mild, moderate, severe and profound learning disabilities. For the purpose of describing the study, I grouped people together as follows:

- People with mild and moderate learning disabilities – likely to result in learning difficulties in school and possible developmental delays in childhood; most can learn to develop some degree of independence, acquire adequate communication skills, and will be able to live and work in the community with varying levels of support; many will be able to maintain good social relationships.
- People with severe and profound learning disabilities – likely to result in continuous need for support, and possible severe limitations in self-care, continence, communication and mobility.

(World Health Organisation 1992)

There were seven participants with mild/moderate learning disabilities, who had good or reasonable verbal comprehension and ability (Sally, Amanda, John, Pauline, Richard, Lily and Vincent); and six with severe/profound learning disabilities, who had no or very limited verbal ability (Nick, Pete, Ben, Dimas, Marion and Ursula).

The Department of Health (2001a) estimates that there are around 145,000 adults with severe and profound learning disabilities in England,

and almost ten times as many people with mild and moderate learning disabilities: some 1.2 million people. Emerson and Hatton (2008) estimate that there are 177,000 known adult users of learning disability services in England.

Ethnographic methods

Finding a good way to answer the question 'What is it like for people with learning disabilities to have cancer?' needed some thought. The sample included people who spoke eloquently, but also people who couldn't tell me about their experiences. People with severe communication difficulties, particularly those with the most severe cognitive impairments, have been even more excluded from research participation than those who could, with support if needed, take part in interview- or questionnaire-based research. To gain in-depth insights, and to accommodate the wide range of abilities and needs of the study population, I adopted an ethnographic methodology.

Ethnography has its roots in anthropology, and typically involves prolonged periods of participant observation. In a nutshell, the ethnographer tries to understand the world of the population under study, by becoming part of that world. To this end, I spent a lot of time (over 250 hours in total) in the company of the participants. Of course, as Atkinson *et al.* (2001) point out:

> Participant observation alone would normally result in strange and unnatural behaviour were the observer not to talk to his or her hosts, so turning them into informants or 'co-researchers'. Hence, conversations and interviews are often indistinguishable from other forms of interaction and dialogue in field research settings... In principle, indeed, the ethnographer may find herself or himself drawing on a very diverse repertoire of research techniques. (Atkinson *et al.* 2001, p.5)

The defining characteristic of ethnography is that, whatever the range of data collection techniques, it remains firmly rooted in first-hand exploration of research settings – in this case, the social settings of the participants.

My most important goal was to be with the participants and to experience, in some small way, what they experienced. It was important to give them the message that it was not my role to 'do' anything for them, that I was not in any position of responsibility, but was simply there because I was interested in their lives. Even those who could not understand the purpose of the study, or the meaning of my presence, eventually understood that I was there for *them*. Nick Ballard, who had severe learning disabilities, no hearing and no speech, seemed somewhat confused when I first turned up at his home, having only seen me at his day centre so far. What on earth was I doing in his house? Day centre staff never visited him at home. It wasn't until I also appeared at his hospital appointments and, later, at the side of his hospital bed that he began to greet me with enthusiasm, communicated more with me and clearly enjoyed my visits.

The advantage of using ethnographic methodologies was that this allowed me to explore people's experiences from a variety of angles. Apart from talking to and spending time with the participants, I also spoke with their families, social care staff, day care staff, doctors and nurses, listening to their views, questions and concerns. I attended review meetings, studied personal and medical files, and occasionally gave feedback sessions to staff after someone had died, providing an opportunity for shared reflection. I attended seven funerals, and returned to visit staff or relatives after people had died, sometimes months or even a few years later. After the data collection period had ended, I kept in contact with some surviving participants and a number of the bereaved families and carers; those contacts, too, have been incorporated in this book.

It was not possible, desirable or ethically sound to remain detached and impartial. As a participant observer, I was not there simply to watch and listen, but to take part in people's lives if appropriate. I helped staff out by driving someone home from a hospital appointment. I helped participants to get comfortable in bed and held their hand when they were frightened, sad or lonely. I hugged their distressed families and sometimes cried with them. I acted as a sounding board for staff and gave them directions or feedback when they were unsure about the care they provided. I always suggested that they talk to the relevant professionals involved in the person's care, and was careful not to undermine other people's roles, but I could not deny the carers my professional expertise at times when it was clearly needed. Families and care staff knew that I had worked as a hospice nurse for many years, and that I had managed a home for people with severe learning disabilities. They often looked to me for support.

When Lily Lamb's support workers struggled to cope with Lily's pain, they telephoned their hospice nurse for help, but they also asked me for immediate advice. Pete Carpenter's carers wanted me to talk to them about Pete's physical deterioration. When people were dying, I reassured their families and carers in the same way I would have done if I had been their palliative care nurse. I believe it would have been unethical to withhold my expertise at these times.

Similarly, I answered the questions of doctors and nurses if I felt that my help would benefit the person's care. When Lily was admitted to the hospice, the nurses asked me for advice on how to communicate with her, and recorded that advice in her notes.

There were huge variations in the length of time the participants were involved. The average length of involvement (both mean and median) was seven months, but at one end of the spectrum, Dimas Ferreira died on the evening of the day I first met him. At the other end, I visited Vincent Sweeney regularly for two years. As a result, some participants' stories emerged more comprehensively than others'. It was perhaps more difficult to get a clear sense of people's lives, and the meaning of their death, if I had not met them before they were so ill that their usual communication methods had changed. In those cases, I had to rely less on direct talking with and observing of the participants, and more on reports from families and other carers in trying to understand the participants' lives.

Communication methods inevitably shaped the data collection. Some people, including John Davies, Vincent Sweeney and Amanda Cresswell, talked eloquently and at great length. They tended to see my visits as interviews, and wanted to use the time to tell me as much as possible about their experiences. It was more difficult to act as an observer with them; they did not expect or even want me to just 'hang out'. These visits rarely lasted more than an hour, and sometimes much less than that; it was as much talking as I could comfortably keep in my brain, and as much as both the participant and myself could cope with. Richard Horwood, for example, often did not want to meet me for longer than 20 minutes. He lacked the energy, and although he was clearly keen to be involved in the study, he did not want to dwell on his life or his cancer for longer than that.

It was more difficult to understand the meaning of the experiences of people who lacked verbal communication skills, and I tended to spend more time with them, usually a couple of hours at varying times each week, in different settings if possible. Crucially, though, I wrote down not only my conversations with the participants, but also my observations about their social environments and their interactions with others. In most cases, the focus of my visits changed as I got to know the participants and their carers, from what may have felt like a formal 'interview' to a more informal, friendly and supportive presence. At first, I might ask my participants to tell me about their illness and their lives. As time progressed, people began to ask me about my work and my children; people with learning disabilities and their carers asked me to help out with some of the care needs; and it often became more comfortable for all of us just to sit in silence. It felt like a two-way relationship, and this enabled me to gain a much greater depth of understanding. I was happy to give out my home phone number to everyone involved in the study, which people have used but never abused. It was essential that I was kept informed of people's progress. The personal relationships I had built meant that I was informed and able to sit at Lily Lamb's death bed on a Sunday afternoon. I didn't mind being telephoned by the brother of John Davies one Easter Sunday, months after John's death, telling me that their mother had now also died – I attended her funeral, too. As John's brother said, 'Of course you can come to Mum's funeral. You're part of it now.'

Being part of it: that was the aim and the essence of the data collection. It was the gradual realisation of the responsibility involved in becoming 'part of it', a responsibility to do justice to the generosity and courage of the participants and the people around them in sharing their lives with me – all the way to the time of their deaths and beyond – that made me decide to write this book.

Recruiting the participants

The in-depth qualitative investigation of people's experiences was a time-consuming task, and 13 people were as many as I could manage in the given time, both practically and emotionally. The number of participants partly depended on the length of time someone was involved in the study. There were around four participants at any one time, and I could only see a new participant if another had died or if, after months of intensive visiting, I could reduce the frequency of visits. After two years, a clear picture began to emerge. Although every person's experience was unique, there were certain aspects that formed a common thread, and the last three participants revealed no new themes.

Nine participants were recruited through personal contacts with health professionals, usually through conferences about palliative care or learning disabilities. The other four participants came through a call on a learning disability internet forum. The first seven participants were selected simply because I heard about them and it was convenient to include them (convenience sampling). The final six were specifically chosen because I wanted to explore emerging concepts, and to ensure a wide range of contexts and experiences (theoretical sampling) (Strauss and Corbin 1998).

The remit of the Veronica Project was that people with cancer at any stage could be included, but it proved difficult to recruit people with learning disabilities who were newly diagnosed with cancer. The information and consent process was usually lengthy, and by the time these were completed, the person had either already gone through the cancer treatments, or had unexpectedly died.

Most participants were terminally ill. It became clear that the in-depth study of real-life experiences was particularly suitable for people whose health status was changing, and less useful when people's cancer was in remission and no longer dominated their lives. Themes around dying began to emerge. The focus of the Veronica Project gradually shifted from 'living with cancer' to 'dying with cancer'.

I was never short of suitable participants. At one stage I had more than I could cope with. However, it could be difficult to find the wide range of participants that I had hoped for. Most participants were referred to me through a health or social care professional, and this meant that they were all using certain services. Seven of the 13 participants lived in a staffed residential care home; however, in England only 15 per cent of all people with learning disabilities live in a residential care home. Most adults with learning disabilities live at home with their families (55% with a parent, and 12% with other relatives) (Emerson and Hatton 2008). Many of these don't have any outside support. They are under-represented in this book. Also under-represented are those whose residential care staff lacked the support of outside agencies, like palliative care teams or community learning disability teams.

Inclusion in the study usually depended on the goodwill of 'gatekeepers', mostly social care staff, who had to be willing to help the person with learning disabilities consent to and take part in the study. In practice, this meant that the staff had to be prepared to think and talk about cancer, even if the people with learning disabilities themselves did not know the truth about their illness. In some situations, this just seemed too much for the staff. The manager of one home, where a resident had just been diagnosed with terminal cancer, expressed her reasons for not allowing me access very clearly:

> 'I am up to my ears at the moment, trying to sort it all out, trying to support her and make her as comfortable as possible. So I'm not really interested in research at the moment, I can't take that on as well as everything else... I don't want to alarm her. I don't want her to have another new face. She would get quite panicky if she knew something was happening to her.'

It was a pity that I couldn't include people whose carers were so evidently stressed; but this home manager's reasons were understandable and entirely valid.

It was not a prerequisite for the study described in this book that people knew they had cancer. Indeed, I often explained to concerned staff that I also wanted to learn from the experiences of participants who had not been told. It may be that this helped recruitment. There is, however, probably an over-representation of people who knew that they had cancer.

Another challenge of recruitment was the very nature of the illness itself. Many people with learning disabilities are diagnosed late, and time was often of the essence. Information and consent procedures could take weeks, particularly for those who lacked capacity to understand and consent to the study, as it involved conversations with many parties, including social care staff and relatives. Sometimes staff suggested that I wait until 'things settled down' with the person. I learned to be gently persistent, knowing that things would probably never settle down – in fact, they were invited into the study precisely because things were *not* settled down. On two occasions, the person died before I could start visiting. In the case of Dimas Ferreira, consent procedures took six weeks; he died in the evening of my first meeting with him.

Writing field notes

The data consisted of over 1500 pages of closely typed field notes. After each visit, I would spend several hours writing down as much as I could remember. In the field notes, I recorded exactly what I had observed in as much detail as I could remember. I wrote down what happened, how people looked, what they wore, what they did, how they behaved, how they interacted, what they said, what silences there were. I wrote down how all this made me feel, what I was thinking during the silences, how I reacted emotionally to what was happening.

Not using a tape recorder meant that I could be flexible, move around, talk to people whenever and wherever seemed relevant. The disadvantage was that there are inevitable inaccuracies in my recorded field notes, with sentences that are often paraphrased rather than written down verbatim. I trained myself to remember as much as I could. Occasionally, if I wanted to remember something word for word, I would go somewhere private (usually the toilet!) and write it down on a small notepad. On the way home, I spoke into a tape recorder, trying in particular to remember people's vocabulary, what they had said and how they had said it.

Reading the field notes two years after individuals died, I instantly conjured up the way they looked and behaved in my mind's eye; I heard their voices in my mind's ear, in a way that simply thinking about them could no longer do. This reassured me that I had captured them fairly accurately, and that my method of remembering and writing had been reasonably effective. After I sent extracts from the draft of this book to Sarah, Marion Prentice's sister, she rang me and said, 'When I read it, I remembered saying all those things. You have put it exactly as I said it, word for word.' Someone else wrote to me, 'You have got the wording spot on.'

One day, when I thought the tape recorder was turned on as I was listening to Amanda Cresswell, I realised after ten minutes that it was not working. When it came to writing field notes, I could not remember at all what had been said during those ten minutes. I could remember very clearly the half hour of conversation leading up it, but I had obviously concentrated less on the content of the 'taped' conversation, believing that there was no need – it would all be neatly transcribed.

This showed me that I had trained myself rather effectively in the art of looking and listening intently, and that this had probably not only served the stated purpose of writing accurate field notes, but had also taught me to listen well. I could never allow myself to switch off and let my mind wander, or even to think about the next thing I was going to say, because that would distract me from hearing what was happening. If I did switch off, that in itself would be worth writing down and was a cause for later contemplation. What was it in this situation that I could not manage to stay with? Was it all too much for me at that moment, and did I need extra support or supervision, or simply a break from data collection? Or was it actually too boring, too unimportant, maybe even too painful in my eyes, that I had to shield them? And if that was so, what did that mean for the persons involved, who could not shield their eyes?

Now, I wonder whether it might have been beneficial in my past clinical roles as a nurse to have the attributes of an ethnographic researcher, someone whose aim it is to see the world from the other person's perspective, trying not only to look but to see, not only to listen but to hear.

For further details on how field notes are used in ethnographic research, and how conversations can be recorded, see Emerson, Fretz and Shaw (2001).

Data analysis

The field notes were analysed not only by myself, but also by four colleagues. They had followed people's stories as I had been sharing them, back in the office. We picked out emerging themes as I went along, and I fed those themes back into the data collection, looking for similarities and differences, and occasionally asking participants and their carers whether my findings with other participants rang bells for them. Sometimes they identified strongly, and sometimes they didn't, explaining why things were different for them. This way of collecting and analysing data at the same time followed the principles of Grounded Theory (Strauss and Corbin 1998).

At the end of the data collection period, Jane Bernal, a psychiatrist working with people with learning disabilities who had been involved with the Veronica Project from the beginning, read all my field notes one weekend – all 1500 pages. By now, I had immersed myself into these field notes, and had spent months trying to make sense of them. It was invaluable that there was someone else who knew exactly what had happened with all the participants. At the end of that weekend, Jane wrote: 'I knew what you were doing, and yet I didn't. I certainly did not realise the size and richness of the task.' She analysed the notes independently, before I gave her my own interpretation. We spent many hours talking about the data, comparing our interpretations and slowly moving towards what we felt was the essence of the findings.

I then turned the field notes into 13 comprehensive stories, putting in everything I felt was relevant, including large sections of the original field notes. I gave the stories to Sheila Hollins (professor of learning disability), Jane Hubert (social anthropologist) and Gary Butler (training and research advisor). Unaware of the themes Jane Bernal and I had pulled out, they each generated their own list of themes and sub-themes.

I supported Gary (who has learning disabilities himself) to do this by noting down exactly what his comments were as he read the stories out loud, which sections left him laughing, feeling sad, or (in his own words) 'fuming'. At the end of each story, I asked him what had struck him most, what was important, and whether anything in the story reminded him of something else. Sometimes, he was reminded of other participants' stories he read earlier; often, he was reminded of his own life.

And that was true for all of us. The aspects of people's stories that struck us most, or maybe made us most upset, were often aspects that somehow resonated with our own professional or personal lives. We had to be aware of our own researcher bias.

Researcher bias

My field notes were inevitably coloured by my personal and professional background, as a palliative care nurse, a learning disability nurse, a mother of young children, and a friend of a number of people with learning disabilities.

I was shocked by the social and emotional deprivation of some of the places where people with learning disabilities lived and spent their daytime hours, because it had been decades since I had been confronted with such deprivation (in the long-stay institutions of the Netherlands in the 1980s), and I had perhaps believed that it no longer existed. Researchers with more recent clinical experience in learning disability services may have described this aspect of people's lives in less vivid ways; they may have been less shocked.

Someone with little or no experience of terminal illness may have been more shocked by the painful and relentless process of physical deterioration as someone approaches death. Having seen hundreds of people die, I did not note this in the same way. What I did note were those instances where end-of-life support, and in particular symptom control, did not match up to the high palliative care standards I had been trained in. I interpreted some subtle behavioural indicators as possible physical pain, where a different researcher might have interpreted them as emotional distress.

Gary, whose life experience included living in a staffed residential care home before moving on to live in his own flat, recognised the truth of people's dependent lives and the importance of 'genuine' carers, people who really care about you and don't just treat you as their job. This helped to develop the theme of the importance of carers who are warm and loving.

Sheila, who is not only a distinguished professor and psychiatrist but also the mother of an adult son with learning disabilities – and who, at the time of analysis, was involved in the independent inquiry which investigated discrimination of people with learning disabilities in hospitals

(Michael 2008) – saw confirmation of the crucial place of the family, and pointed out instances of discriminatory practice.

Jane Hubert, the anthropologist, consistently emphasised the importance of trying to look at these stories through people's own eyes.

Jane Bernal was interested in several emerging themes and helped them develop, including dependence, social identity, truth-telling and remembrance. Her past experience as a member of a research ethics committee supported a strong focus on the ethical aspects of the Veronica Project.

It was invaluable to see, through our combined analyses, where our biases lay; but, more importantly, it was invaluable to see that despite all these biases and differences in focus, our analysis was fundamentally the same. All of us (including Gary) had distilled the same overall themes. These are the themes that have shaped this book. I must acknowledge the contribution of these four colleagues, and in particular the influence and guidance of Jane Bernal in the writing of this book.

I recommend that readers examine their own biases, too, and keep doing so when they are personally involved in the support of someone with learning disabilities who has cancer and/or is dying. The aspects of people's lives, illness and care we experience as poignant, difficult or uplifting may well be influenced by our own stories, maybe even our own (sometimes unacknowledged) losses. It is good to know what gives us the strength and inspiration to be with a person with learning disabilities at such a difficult time; it is also good to know what makes it too unbearable for us. Crucially, being aware of our own biases can help us to set them aside and to try to see the world from another person's point of view.

Some of our findings came as no surprise, and confirmed anecdotal clinical experience as well as the literature. Some themes (like 'truth-telling and understanding' and 'inexperienced carers') were evident right from the start. However, the depth of understanding of these themes was new; and some themes only became evident later (for example, 'resilience'). As an example of how the close analysis of 13 people's cancer experiences can bring to light certain important aspects, I quote Jane Bernal, who wrote after reading the field notes:

> 'Communication is an enormous issue for people with learning disabilities. In this work I am struck by the fact that it is not just medical jargon, speech, sensory and cognitive impairments that get in the way, but the fact that people with learning disabilities have often learned to hide their pain and have few expectations that they will be heard. I expected the doctors not to be able

> to speak English, only doctorish, and they did. I expected the information giving to be poor, and it was. I expected non-learning disabilities staff to be unsure whether a person was in pain, and they were. All these are well reported in the literature and your work confirms this. The extent to which some people hide their pain, covering it with a jolly smile, is less expected.'

Ethical issues

A study like this, involving people with learning disabilities who are highly vulnerable, raises a number of ethical issues. Including people with learning disabilities in research is increasingly recognised as important, by people with learning disabilities themselves as well as academics (Department of Health 2006; Gilbert 2006; Walmsley 2004). Although research which includes people with learning disabilities as active participants is now fairly common, their inclusion in research around sensitive topics remains controversial (Lindop 2006). There are difficult questions about consent and the possibility to inflict harm. Inclusive research about cancer, death and dying remains largely uncharted territory. At the start of the work, I found only two published studies that included interviews with people with intellectual disabilities (Brown *et al.* 2002; Todd 2004).

There has been a debate within palliative care research generally about whether it is ethical for a vulnerable population of people who are dying to be included in research at all, given that there may be no benefit to compensate the loss of their already limited time and energy (Addington-Hall 2002; Wilkie 2001). Increasingly, it is recognised that participation in research can be an empowering experience for people who are terminally ill, providing an opportunity to make a final valuable contribution (Hopkinson and Wright 2005; Terry *et al.* 2006). The question is less stark for patients who have cancer and are not terminally ill, but ethical issues remain about the demands research participation could place on very ill and vulnerable patients.

However, in order to provide sensitive, appropriate and evidence-based support for people who have cancer and/or are terminally ill, a sound body of research is needed. We need to know how the illness is experienced, what helps, what hinders, how we can best support people. The question, therefore, was not *if* we should include people with learning disabilities in the study, but *how*. An important and recurrent finding from our other studies has been that it is possible for people with intellectual disabilities to contribute to an expansion of knowledge through participation in research, even when that involves highly sensitive topics like cancer, death and dying (Tuffrey-Wijne *et al.* 2006; Tuffrey-Wijne *et al.* 2007). This echoed the findings of Todd, who reported that the people with intellectual disabilities he interviewed on the topic of death 'turned out to be more relaxed and eager to talk about this issue than I had anticipated' (Todd 2004, p.13). Our own experience of research participants with learning disabilities suggests that they are enthusiastic, not only because of the empowering experience of being listened to, but also because of an understanding that through participation they could make a contribution that would help their peers.

The study was approved by the South East Multi-Centre Ethics Committee (COREC) in 2005 (reference number 05/MRE01/29). A research advisory group was set up and met twice a year, to provide guidance on future data collection and, in particular, to safeguard ethical standards. As well as the four colleagues who helped with data analysis, the group included two further members with learning disabilities, a specialist cancer nurse, a palliative care consultant, a representative from the Down's Syndrome Association, and representatives from three providers of residential care for people with learning disabilities: United Response, The Home Farm Trust and McIntyre Care.

Capacity to consent

The questions of how to obtain consent, how to provide accessible study information, and how to proceed if participants lack capacity to understand such information, are of crucial importance. I was rightly asked about this by the Research Ethics Committee, by potential participants' carers, and by the people with learning disabilities on the research advisory group.

Some people in our study not only lacked capacity to understand the concept of a research study, but they also did not know they had cancer. The study was conducted before the Mental Capacity Act 2005 passed into English Law (Department for Constitutional Affairs 2007). This new legal framework requires researchers to identify and consult someone who is not a professional carer for the participants; the participant must be withdrawn from the study if this 'advocate' feels he or she does not wish to take part. In our study, proxy assent was sought from a main carer or relative. We adopted the principle of 'process consent' (Department of Health 2001b), giving continuous attention to the question of whether the participant seemed happy to engage with the researcher. At times, this meant cutting short a planned data collection visit.

I learned to take different cues from each participant. I would ask Sally Burnett whether she wanted me to go home or stay a bit longer, and the fact that she did not always answer in the same way probably meant that she was truthful. When Richard Horwood asked politely, 'When is your train?' it meant that he wanted me to go and catch it as soon as possible. Lily Lamb was always very pleased to see me, but would sometimes suddenly say 'See you next week,' which was code for 'I've had enough.' John Davies indicated that he was tired of talking by changing the subject and asking me how my children were; and once or twice he was so fed up with life that he didn't want to see me. There were also a number of occasions where someone was not at home at the agreed time; it is impossible to say whether this was due to a poor memory and sense of time, or an unspoken wish to avoid seeing the researcher on that particular day. I had to learn to cope cheerfully with the waste of a three-hour round trip as part and parcel of the research process.

One can question whether it can ever be ethical to include ill and vulnerable people in a study about cancer, if they can have no idea about the purpose of the study. Is it ethical to include them in what is arguably an intrusive study, allowing a researcher access to their lives, if they cannot give their consent? However, the importance of understanding the experiences of those who lacked capacity to understand the reason for the researcher's presence, and of those who were unaware of their diagnosis, justified their inclusion. In fact, it could also be argued that it is unethical to exclude people with more severe learning disabilities from studies that could provide insight into their experiences and help to shape sensitive care in the future. The Research Ethics Committee agreed, but wanted to be explicitly reassured that we would not reveal any information to the participants about their diagnosis or prognosis. Carers, too, wanted this reassurance. We produced two different versions of the study information sheet: one mentioned 'cancer', the other simply 'illness'.

There was an unexpected twist to the possibility of researchers revealing information to participants when a nurse who previewed the study information sheet looked concerned. When I asked her whether this was because the person didn't know he had cancer, she replied, 'Oh, he knows that – but I'm not sure he knows he has learning disabilities!'

Anonymity

We were asking participants to share deeply personal experiences. Some of them knew their stories would be published. They seemed to find the realisation that what they had gone through could be of importance to the outside world highly empowering. Whilst some sought reassurance that I would keep their situation confidential ('Don't put my name in that book!'), two participants, John Davies and Amanda Cresswell, were very clear that they wanted to stand up and 'own' their stories.

An important feature of qualitative research with people with learning disabilities is to make their stories heard, to give voice to a previously silenced group. The need to anonymise the data was sometimes very difficult to explain. Anticipating that some participants might strongly object to – or even be offended by – having their stories anonymised, the research protocol included the possibility of foregoing anonymity. The possible use of people's own name was given ethical approval; John and Amanda each published their stories in their own words (Cresswell and Tuffrey-Wijne 2008; Tuffrey-Wijne and Davies 2007).

The literature on ethical issues in qualitative research places a heavy emphasis on the need to protect participants from harm, typically through assuring confidentiality (Baez 2002). However, some have argued that research participants' autonomous choice to waive their right to confidentiality should be seriously considered, with careful examination of the reasons for refusing the participant such a choice, as well as the implications of allowing it (Giordano *et al.* 2007).

In practice, granting a wish to be identified was not an easy decision and caused considerable debate, both with John and Amanda and within the research team. Stepping out of anonymity would also identify people's families and carers, and the participants had to understand the implications of this. Amanda took matters into her own hands by telephoning the editors of a journal with the offer to submit her written story; I could not deny her the right to be the author of that story. John spent many months considering, trying to understand what forgoing anonymity might mean for his family, until his family gave him the reassurance that they supported his wishes.

However, whilst 'being named' has undoubtedly added poignancy and power to John's story, there were unexpected ethical complications. Aspects of the care John and his family received in the weeks leading up to and immediately after his death, after his story went to press, were so shocking that I wrote a formal letter of complaint to the nursing home. This is part of the research findings, but I now realise that the decision to identify John potentially means that *everyone* involved in his situation could potentially be identified, even if they hadn't formally agreed to this. Is that ethically sound?

Lack of anonymity could affect the rigor of the study. I would probably have written in more detail about John and his family, and about the research team's analysis of his life, illness and death, if he had been anonymous. Researchers may feel less free to construct theory from stories that are so clearly owned by those who told them. Accommodating participants' right to refuse anonymity could therefore undermine the ultimate research objective.

Despite these possibilities, the research team believed that it was ethically justified to give highly vulnerable people an opportunity to leave the legacy they so desperately wanted. Being able to do this gave their illness meaning and helped them to move on in different ways: to rebuild life or to accept death. It did not seem ethical to deny people this opportunity.

Observation of sub-optimal care

At times I witnessed sub-optimal care, and this raised different ethical issues. At what point should I step out of my neutral role and influence the situation? The research protocol stated that the researcher could intervene if a (lack of) care and support seemed detrimental to the participant's well-being; and that before intervening, the researcher should seek guidance from certain members of the research advisory group who had agreed to act as an ethics sub-committee. Intervention by the researcher would inevitably lead to a change in the person's situation and would therefore affect the data collected. However, we agreed it was unethical to observe seriously inadequate care without intervention: the welfare of the participant had to come before the needs of the researchers.

In practice, this was not always straightforward. When is care sub-optimal? There were many occasions where I observed practice that may not have been optimal, but that did not warrant intervention. Rather, these observations were simply part of the findings. Examples include participants being patronised or ignored by hospital staff, or participants' wishes not being acted on by support workers.

There were a few occasions when, having consulted the research advisory group, I intervened. For example, Nick Ballard clearly and consistently indicated that he was in pain, but his home manager did not want to give him regular analgesia. My suggestions to get a palliative care review were not followed up. I became concerned when Nick began to lose his balance, a possible sign of spinal cord compression which could lead to irreversible paralysis and can be prevented by prompt treatment. After seeking advice from the palliative care consultant on the research advisory group, I spoke of my concerns to the home manager and to Nick's hospital medical team.

An observation of abusive behaviour was more challenging. Chapter 6 gives details of abuse suffered by Ursula Smith at the hands of a support worker in her residential care home. I could not report this immediately, as the home manager was absent. I consulted the research advisory group and reported the incident to the home manager some days later, insisting on a report to social services under the 'Protection of Vulnerable Adults' structure. The support worker was suspended, the incident was investigated, and this contributed to the support worker's decision to leave her employment. On reflection, I felt that I should have intervened immediately, but such decisions can be difficult, particularly as a researcher's role is usually explicitly *not* to intervene. In future research protocols, I will now include the clause that the researcher may intervene without consulting the research advisory group if he/she believes that the participant is at immediate risk from harm, working on the principle that it is unethical not to intervene when observing harmful situations.

The researcher–participant relationship

Research participants with learning disabilities are unlikely to be familiar with the role of the researcher, and this can be of particular significance in ethnographic research, where the risk of intrusion is great. Stalker (1998) highlights the concern that the researcher will be unable to meet expectations of continuing friendship. Angrosino (2004) warns that the engagement of the participant observer may be especially delicate as people with learning disabilities may have limited experience with friendships, and may have emotional needs for which the researcher is not fully prepared.

Like Booth and Booth (1994b) in their study of parents who have learning disabilities, I treated rapport as a two-way process, and was happy to share details of my own life with the participants when asked. I also tried to be as clear and honest as possible about my involvement and its limitations, and to keep appointments and promises. The initial research protocol stipulated an involvement of around four months. However, as the study progressed, that seemed not only too short to collect all the relevant data; it also seemed unethical to withdraw what had become, in many cases, a supportive presence. While I was always aware that as a researcher I was not a therapist or indeed a friend in the usual sense, with some people it was clear that I could not suddenly end the relationship. Booth and Booth state that 'social researchers using biographical methods with vulnerable groups must be prepared to live up to this commitment or risk their field relationship becoming exploitative' (Booth and Booth 1994a, p.419). With some participants, I developed close bonds that lasted beyond death. I still miss them.

Coping with the Veronica Project

I started the work with what was, looking back, a certain naivety. Colleagues questioned how I would cope, but I responded that I would be fine, and initially didn't take up the offer of personal supervision. I thought that my experience as a hospice nurse had prepared me well. There had been times in the hospice when several of my patients died in the same week. Whilst I hope that the support I gave them was warm and genuine, I rarely took my concerns about these patients home with me. Nurses working with dying patients somehow learn to cope with the intense emotions they are confronted with on a daily basis, the physical and emotional pain of the patients, the distress of the families. They have the support of their colleagues, who are always ready to talk things through in the office; and they know their boundaries. Of course, there were some patients and families that affected me and stayed with me; but generally, I learned to put patients' distress behind me very quickly. I had to be able to hold a dying patient's hand and sit with a distraught family in one room, and moments later join another family in the next room, rejoicing together in how well the patient is today.

I genuinely thought that I didn't need much support in managing the emotional impact of the study. I could cope with death and dying. Having lived with people with learning disabilities for many years, I also thought I could cope with being close to the people in the study – but I wasn't prepared for the effect of trying to understand the experiences of people with learning disabilities from the inside. Soon, I discovered that the protective mechanisms that had helped me as a nurse were of little use in my role as an ethnographic researcher; in fact, it was essential to strip away the barriers clinicians use to make it possible to witness other people's agony.

The fact that I was *not* a palliative care nurse for my participants made a crucial difference. I was not there to sort things out, but simply to listen; my only reason for spending time with them was that I was interested in their story, and I wanted to know what it was like to be in their shoes. This could be difficult, sometimes unbearably so; not being able to step in and help, and not being able to walk away to the next patient when things were too painful, was a considerable challenge. It also turned out to be a precious gift. My role was to bear witness, no more and no less; simply being there with people, week after week, month after month, gave them a powerful message that their lives mattered, and they responded with trust and generosity. I saw their vulnerability and their strength, and unlike my relationships with my hospice patients, I could not leave these behind when I went home. They became part of my life; I wrote about them and thought about them very deeply. After a one-hour session, I would be writing for several hours, often late at night, and I would spend many weeks and months – and, as it turned out during the final analysis, even years – thinking about the lives of the people I had been with.

The death of John Davies, one year into the study, was an emotional turning point. He was the fourth participant to die, and it was devastating. The cumulative effect of living with the intense emotions and grief of John, his family, and all the other people with learning disabilities, carers and families took its toll. A fifth participant died a week later; in that same week, I also attended the funeral of a personal friend who had learning disabilities. It felt like too many funerals and too much grief, and I had to take several months off from collecting data.

It finally became clear to me that this kind of work could not be done without strong support and excellent supervision, and I was fortunate that I had access to both. I am indebted to the combined support of my colleagues and superiors, Sheila Hollins, Jane Bernal and Jane Hubert. They noticed when I wasn't coping well and helped me back on track. I am also deeply grateful for the excellent personal supervision offered by Valerie Sinason and Dorothy Judd, both psychotherapists with great warmth and understanding. I now know that good supervision is an ethical issue too. This includes not only work supervision around the practical and analytical aspects of the study, but also personal supervision – someone to help you reflect on your own emotions. Without such support, the potential for harm to the participants and the researcher is just too great. As a researcher it is important to have someone alongside you, looking over your shoulder and talking things through, regardless of how senior you are.

I look back on the Veronica Project as one of the greatest challenges and one of the greatest privileges of my career. To be allowed, indeed required, to spend time with people at such a crucial and profound time in their lives, and to be able to take plenty of time to think about them and to write their stories, has changed the way I look at people. I am sure this will benefit the people I will work with in the future. Now, I meet people and wonder... Who are you? What is *your* story? What has your life been like? What has made you who you are today? What matters most to you? I am deeply grateful to all the people in this book for making me ask those questions.

Endnotes

Chapter 1: Three Stories

1. Makaton is a communication system where key words in the spoken language are supported by signs taken from British Sign Language. It is used by many people with learning disabilities in the UK.
2. One of these women was Ursula Smith, who became a participant in the Veronica Project six months after Nick died.
3. Cystoscopy: examining and treating the inside of the bladder with the help of a camera on a long tube.
4. Urostomy bag: a bag that is fixed over a surgically made opening in the skin, usually on the stomach. Urine is led through the opening into the bag.
5. Morphine is usually the drug of choice for cancer pain, and it is rare for cancer patients to become addicted to it.
6. Syringe driver: a small portable machine, linking a syringe to a needle under the skin, giving a continuous infusion of drugs.

Chapter 2: Diagnosis and Treatment

7. Bronchoscopy: looking into the lungs with a camera at the end of a tube.

Chapter 3: Truth-telling and Understanding

8. Vincent died almost two years later, just as I was writing this chapter.
9. Colostomy bag: a colostomy is a surgical procedure where the colon (part of the bowels) is cut and brought through the abdomen, creating an artificial opening; the faeces are collected in a pouch, the colostomy bag, which is attached to the opening. Sally lived with her colostomy for over five years, changing the bag every day.
10. Supra-pubic catheter: a tube going straight into the bladder through a hole made in the skin of the abdomen, connected to a bag to drain urine.

Chapter 6: Dependent Lives

11. Vincent was suspicious of anyone talking about him behind his back, and hated people passing on to others what he had told them in confidence. However, he always knew that I would write about him in a book. I explained to him that

although I wouldn't use his real name, his family and nurses would recognise him in my writing. I asked him whether there was anything he wanted me to keep out of this book, giving him examples of sensitive information, such as his failure to take his medication or details of abuse suffered when he was young. He gave his explicit permission to publish everything he told me.

Resources

Useful reading

Books Beyond Words

Books Beyond Words is a series of picture books that has been developed to make communicating easier for people with learning disabilities, and to enable discussion about difficult topics. The pictures are designed to help readers make sense of what is happening to them, and help them to ask questions or share their concerns. Supporting text and guidelines are also provided for carers, supporters and professionals. Published by RCPsych/St George's University of London. Available from www.rcpsych.ac.uk/publications/booksbeyondwords.aspx

Selected useful titles in the Books Beyond Words series

Am I Going to Die? *by Sheila Hollins and Irene Tuffrey-Wijne (2009)*
This book is based on the findings of the Veronica Project. It tells the story of a man who has learning disabilities and who is dying. The pictures follow him in his illness and his final days.

Getting On With Cancer *by Veronica Donaghey, Jane Bernal, Irene Tuffrey-Wijne and Sheila Hollins (2002)*
This is based on the story of Veronica Donaghey, whom the Veronica Project was named after. The book tells the story of a woman who is diagnosed with cancer, and then has surgery, radiotherapy and chemotherapy. The book ends on a positive note.

When Dad Died *and* **When Mum Died** *both by Sheila Hollins and Lester Sireling (1989)*
These books tell the story of the death of a parent in a simple but moving way.

When Somebody Dies *by Sheila Hollins, Noëlle Blackman and Sandra Dowling (2003)*
This book shows people with learning disabilities that they need not be alone when they feel sad about someone's death, and that talking about it to a friend or to a counsellor can help them get through this difficult time.

Going to the Doctor *by Sheila Hollins, Jane Bernal and Matthew Gregory (1996)*
This book illustrates a variety of experiences which may occur at a GP practice, including having one's ears syringed, a physical examination, a blood test and a blood pressure check.

Going to Out-patients *by Sheila Hollins, Angie Avis and Samantha Cheverton (1998)*
This book explains what happens in outpatient departments, covering tests such as ultrasound, X-ray and hearing test.

Going into Hospital *by Sheila Hollins, Jane Bernal and Matthew Gregory (1998)*
This book explains what happens in hospital, including a planned admission for an operation and an emergency admission.

Looking after my Breasts *by Sheila Hollins and Wendy Perez (2000)*
Designed to support women who are invited for breast screening, including a woman having a mammogram and a woman who demonstrates how to be aware of changes in your own breasts.

Keeping Healthy 'Down Below' *by Sheila Hollins and Jackie Downer (2000)*
Designed to support women who are invited for a smear test.

Other useful titles

Caring for People with Learning Disabilities who are Dying *by Noëlle Blackman and Stuart Todd (2005). Worth Publishing, London.*
A concise, clearly written and practical book full of advice for service managers and staff working in learning disability services.

Palliative Care for People with Learning Disabilities *edited by Sue Read (2006). Quay Books, London.*
The chapters in this book address a range of issues around death, dying and learning disabilities. Aimed at practitioners, service managers and policy makers.

Loss and Learning Disability *by Noëlle Blackman (2003). Worth Publishing, London.*
This book is for care staff, therapists and counsellors working with people with learning disabilities. It talks about how people with learning disabilities can be affected by bereavement. It includes ways to prevent normal grief from becoming a bigger problem and ways of helping people when the grief process 'goes wrong'.

Healthcare for All: Independent Inquiry into Access to Healthcare for People with Learning Disabilities
Led by Sir Jonathan Michael, the independent inquiry (2008) sought to identify the action needed to ensure adults and children with learning disabilities receive appropriate treatment in acute and primary health care in England. The report is available as a PDF from www.iahpld.org.uk. Also available in an easy-read version.

Useful services and organisations

Community teams for people with learning disabilities

These are specialist multidisciplinary health teams that support adults with learning disabilities and their families and carers by assessment, by supporting access to mainstream health care, and by providing a range of clinical interventions. Your GP or social services department should have the details of your local team.

Hospice Information Service (from Help the Hospices)

Website: www.helpthehospices.org.uk/our-services/information-service
Phone: 020 7520 8222
Provides information about hospice care and about locally available hospice and palliative care services.

Macmillan Information Line

Website: www.macmillan.org.uk
Phone: 0808 808 2020
Provides practical, emotional, medical and financial advice for people affected by cancer in general. Also provides information about Macmillan services as well as other cancer organisations and support agencies.

Network for Palliative Care of People with Learning Disabilities

Email: chair@natnetpald.org.uk
Phone: 0797 7260967
Encourages and contributes to the development of good practice in the palliative care of people with learning disabilities, through networking and organising national and regional study days.

Cruse Bereavement Care

Website: www.cruse.org.uk
Email: helpline@cruse.org.uk
Phone: 0844 477 9400
Offers free bereavement counselling, support and information to anyone affected by death (including paid carers).

Respond

Website: www.respond.org.uk
Phone: 0808 808 0700
This organisation supports people with learning disabilities, their carers and professionals around any issue of trauma, including bereavement.

Patient Advice and Liaison Service (PALS)

Website: www.pals.nhs.uk

Mencap Learning Disability Helpline

Phone: 0808 808 111
If you have a problem accessing health care, speak to the Patient Advice and Liason Service (PALS) at your local hospital, or contact the Mencap Learning Disability Helpline.

References

Addington-Hall, J. (2002) 'Research sensitivities to palliative care patients.' *European Journal of Cancer Care 11*, 3, 220–224.

Angrosino, M. (2004) 'Participant Observation and Research on Intellectual Disabilities.' In E. Emerson, C. Hatton, T. Thompson and T. Parmenter (eds) *The International Handbook of Applied Research in Intellectual Disabilities.* Chichester: John Wiley & Sons Ltd.

Atkinson, P., Coffey, A., Delamont, S., Lofland, J. and Lofland, L. (2001) *Handbook of Ethnography.* London: Sage Publications.

Baez, B. (2002) 'Confidentiality in qualitative research: reflections on secrets, power and agency.' *Qualitative Research 2*, 1, 35–58.

Baile, W., Buckman, R., Lenzi, R., Glober, G., Beale, E. and Kudelka, A. (2005) 'SPIKES – a six-step protocol for delivering bad news: application to the patient with cancer.' *The Oncologist 5*, 4, 302–311.

Blackman, N. (2003) *Loss and Learning Disability.* London: Worth Publishing.

Blackman, N. and Todd, S. (2005) *Caring for People with Learning Disabilities who are Dying: A Practical Guide for Carers.* London: Worth Publishing.

Booth, T. and Booth, W. (1994a) 'The use of depth interviewing with vulnerable subjects: lessons from a research study of parents with learning difficulties.' *Social Science and Medicine 39*, 3, 415–424.

Booth, T. and Booth, W. (1994b) *Parenting under Pressure: Mothers and Fathers with Learning Difficulties.* Buckingham: Open University Press.

Brown, H., Burns, S. and Flynn, M. (2002) 'Supporting People through Terminal Illness and Death.' In The Foundation for People with Learning Disabilities (ed.) *Today and Tomorrow: The Report of the Growing Older with Learning Disabilities Programme.* London: Mental Health Foundation.

Buckman, R. (1984) 'Breaking bad news – why is it still so difficult?' *British Medical Journal 288*, 1597–1599.

Chapman, C., Abraham, C., Jenkins, V. and Fallowfield, L. (2003) 'Lay understanding of terms used in cancer consultations.' *Psycho-Oncology 12*, 6, 557–566.

Cooke, L. (1997) 'Cancer and learning disability.' *Journal of Intellectual Disability Research 41*, 4, 312–316.

Cresswell, A. and Tuffrey-Wijne, I. (2008) 'The come back kid: I had cancer, but I got through it.' *British Journal of Learning Disabilities 36*, 3, 152–156.

Department for Constitutional Affairs (2007) *Mental Capacity Act 2005: Code of Practice.* London: The Stationery Office.

Department of Health (2001a) *Valuing People: A New Strategy for Learning Disability for the 21st Century. A White Paper.* London: Department of Health.

Department of Health (2001b) *Seeking Consent: Working with People with Learning Disabilities.* London: Department of Health.

Department of Health (2006) 'Let me in – I'm a researcher!' London: Department of Health.

Doka, K. (1989) *Disenfranchised Grief: Recognizing Hidden Sorrow.* Lanham, MD: Lexington Books.

Donaghey, V., Bernal, J., Tuffrey-Wijne, I. and Hollins, S. (2002) *Getting On With Cancer.* London: Gaskell/St George's Hospital Medical School.

Emerson, E. and Hatton, C. (2008) *People with Learning Disabilities in England.* Lancaster: Centre for Disability Research.

Emerson, R., Fretz, R. and Shaw, L. (2001) 'Participant Observation and Fieldnotes.' In P. Atkinson, A. Coffey, S. Delamont, J. Lofland and L. Lofland (eds) *Handbook of Ethnography*. London: Sage Publications.

Gilbert, T. (2006) 'Involving people with learning disabilities in research: issues and possibilities.' *Health & Social Care in the Community 12*, 4, 298–308.

Giordano, J., O'Reilly, M., Taylor, H. and Dogra, N. (2007) 'Confidentiality and autonomy: the challenge(s) of offering research participants a choice of disclosing their identity.' *Qualitative Health Research 17*, 2, 264–275.

Girgis, A. and Sanson-Fisher, R. (1995) 'Breaking bad news: consensus guidelines for medical practitioners.' *Journal of Clinical Oncology 13*, 99, 2449–2456.

Hogg, J. and Tuffrey-Wijne, I. (2008) 'Cancer and intellectual disabilities: a review of some key contextual issues.' *Journal of Applied Research in Intellectual Disabilities 21*, 6, 509–518.

Hollins, S., Attard, M. T., von Fraunhofer, N., McGuigan, S. and Sedgwick, P. (1998) 'Mortality in people with learning disability: risks, causes, and death certification findings in London.' *Developmental Medicine & Child Neurology 40*, 1, 50–56.

Hopkinson, J. and Wright, D. (2005) 'Seeking new methodology for palliative care research: challenging assumptions about studying people who are approaching the end of life.' *Palliative Medicine 19*, 7, 532–537.

Hubert, J. (2000) 'The Social, Individual and Moral Consequences of Physical Exclusion in Long-stay Institutions.' In J. Hubert (ed.) *Madness, Disability and Social Exclusion: The Archeology and Anthropology of Difference*. London: Routledge.

Hubert, J. and Hollins, S. (2006) 'Men with severe learning disabilities and challenging behaviour in long-stay hospital care: qualitative study.' *British Journal of Psychiatry 188*, 1, 70–74.

Janicki, M., Davidson, P., Henderson, C., McCallion, P. *et al.* (2002) 'Health characteristics and health services utilisation in older adults with intellectual disabilties living in community residences.' *Journal of Intellectual Disability Research 46*, 4, 287–298.

Jenkins, V., Fallowfield, L. and Saul, J. (2001) 'Information needs of patients with cancer: results from a large study in UK cancer centres.' *British Journal of Cancer 84*, 1, 48–51.

Leydon, G., Boulton, M., Moynihan, C., Jones, A. *et al.* (2000) 'Cancer patients' information needs and information seeking behaviour: in depth interview study.' *British Medical Journal 320*, 909–913.

Lindop, E. (2006) 'Research, Palliative Care and Learning Disability.' In S. Read (ed.) *Palliative Care for People with Learning Disabilities*. London: Quay Books.

McEnhill, L. (2004) 'Disability.' In D. Oliviere and B. Monroe (eds) *Death, Dying and Social Differences*. Oxford: Oxford University Press.

McEnhill, L. (2005) 'Specialist Palliative Care Social Work with People who have Learning Disabilities.' In J. Parker (ed.) *Aspects of Social Work and Palliative Care*. London: Quay Books.

McEnhill, L. (2008) 'Breaking bad news of cancer to people with learning disabilities.' *British Journal of Learning Disabilities 36*, 3, 157–164.

Mencap (2007) *Death by Indifference*. London: Mencap.

Michael, J. (2008) *Healthcare for All: Report of the Independent Inquiry into Access to Healthcare for People with Learning Disabilities*. London: Independent Inquiry into Access to Healthcare for People with Learning Disabilities.

Monroe, B. and Oliviere, D. (2007) 'Introduction: Unlocking Resilience in Palliative Care.' In B. Monroe and D. Oliviere (eds) *Resilience in Palliative Care: Achievement in Adversity*. Oxford: Oxford University Press.

Noone, I., Crowe, M., Pillay, I. and O'Keefe, S. (2000) 'Telling the truth about cancer: views of elderly patients and their relatives.' *Irish Medical Journal 93*, 4, 104–105.

Novack, D., Plumer, R., Smith, R., Ochitill, H., Morrow, G. and Bennett, J. (1971) 'Changes in physicians' attitudes toward telling the cancer patient.' *Journal of the American Medical Association 241*, 9, 897–900.

Oken, D. (1961) 'What to tell cancer patients: a study of medical attitudes.' *Journal of the American Medical Association 175*, 13, 1120–1128.

Oswin, M. (1991) *Am I Allowed to Cry? A Study of Bereavement amongst People who have Learning Disabilities*. London: Souvenir Press.

Parliamentary and Health Service Ombudsman (2009) *Six Lives: The Provision of Public Services to People with Learning Disabilities. HC 203 I–VIII.* London: The Stationery Office.

Patja, K., Mölsä, P. and Iivanainen, M. (2001) 'Cause-specific mortality of people with intellectual disability in a population-based, 35-year follow-up study.' *Journal of Intellectual Disability Research 45,* 1, 30–40.

Ptacek, J. and Eberhardt, T. (1996) 'Breaking bad news: a review of the literature.' *Journal of the American Medical Association 276,* 6, 496–502.

Saunders, C. (1960) 'The management of patients in the terminal stage.' *Cancer 6,* 403–417.

Saunders, C. (2006) 'Why I Welcome TV Cameras at the Death Bed.' (First published in the *Daily Mail,* 20 March 1998). In C. Saunders (ed.) *Cecily Saunders: Selected Writings 1958–2004.* Oxford: Oxford University Press.

Seale, C. (1991) 'Communication and awareness about death: a study of a random sample of dying people.' *Social Sciences and Medicine 32,* 8, 943–952.

Sinason, V. (1992) *Mental Handicap and the Human Condition.* London: Free Association Books.

Stalker, K. (1998) 'Some ethical and methodological issues in research with people with learning difficulties.' *Disability & Society 13,* 1, 5–19.

Strauss, A. and Corbin, J. (1998) *Basics of Qualitative Research: Techniques and Procedures for Developing Grounded Theory.* London: Sage Publications.

Terry, W., Olson, G., Ravenscroft, P., Wilss, L. and Boulton-Lewis, G. (2006) 'Hospice patients' views on research in palliative care.' *Internal Medicine Journal 36,* 7, 406–413.

Todd, S. (2002) 'Death does not become us: the absence of death and dying in intellectual disability research.' *Journal of Gerontological Social Work 38,* 1/2, 225–239.

Todd, S. (2004) 'Death counts: the challenge of death and dying in learning disability services.' *Learning Disability Practice 7,* 10, 12–15.

Tuffrey-Wijne, I. (2002) 'The palliative care needs of people with intellectual disabilities: a case study.' *International Journal of Palliative Nursing 8,* 5, 222–232.

Tuffrey-Wijne, I. (2009a) '"Am I a good girl?" Dying people who have a learning disability.' *End of Life Care 3,* 1, 35–39.

Tuffrey-Wijne, I. (2009b) 'The preferred place of care for people who are dying.' *Learning Disability Practice 12,* 6, 16–21.

Tuffrey-Wijne, I. and Davies, J. (2007) 'This is my story: I've got cancer. "The Veronica Project": an ethnographic study of the experiences of people with learning disabilities who have cancer.' *British Journal of Learning Disabilities 35,* 1, 7–11.

Tuffrey-Wijne, I. and McEnhill, L. (2008) 'Communication difficulties and intellectual disability in end-of-life care.' *International Journal of Palliative Nursing 14,* 4, 192–197.

Tuffrey-Wijne, I., Bernal, J., Jones, A., Butler, G. and Hollins, S. (2006) 'People with intellectual disabilities and their need for cancer information.' *European Journal of Oncology Nursing 10,* 2, 106–116.

Tuffrey-Wijne, I., Bernal, J., Butler, G., Hollins, S. and Curfs, L. (2007a) 'Using Nominal Group Technique to investigate the views of people with intellectual disabilities on end-of-life care provision.' *Journal of Advanced Nursing 58,* 1, 80–89.

Tuffrey-Wijne, I., McEnhill, L., Curfs, L. and Hollins, S. (2007b) 'Palliative care provision for people with intellectual disabilities: interviews with specialist palliative care providers in London.' *Palliative Medicine 21,* 6, 493–499.

Tuffrey-Wijne, I., Whelton, R., Curfs, L. and Hollins, S. (2008) 'Palliative care provision for people with intellectual disabilities: a questionnaire survey of specialist palliative care professionals in London.' *Palliative Medicine 22,* 3, 281–290.

Walmsley, J. (2004) 'Involving users with learning difficulties in health improvement: lessons from inclusive learning disability research.' *Nursing Inquiry 11,* 1, 54–64.

Wilkie, P. (2001) 'Ethical Issues in Qualitative Research in Palliative Care.' In D. Field, D. Clark, J. Corner and C. Davis (eds) *Researching Palliative Care.* Buckingham: Open University Press.

World Health Organisation (1992) *ICD–10: The Tenth Revision of the International Statistical Classification of Diseases and Related Health Problems.* Geneva: World Health Organisation.

Young, M. and Cullen, L. (1996) *A Good Death: Conversations with East Londoners.* London: Routledge.

Index

CPSIA information can be obtained at www.ICGtesting.com
Printed in the USA
LVOW05s1500211014

409792LV00001B/351/P

9 781849 050272